THE BEST DAMN
SEX
JOKES,
PERIOD!

OTHER BOOKS EDITED BY JUDY BROWN

The Comedy Thesaurus
Squeaky Clean Comedy
She's So Funny
Jokes to Go
The Funny Pages
Joke Stew
Joke Soup

THE BEST DAMN
SEX
JOKES,
PERIOD!

*Over 550 of the Funniest Dirty Jokes from
the Best Professional Comedians*

Edited by Judy Brown

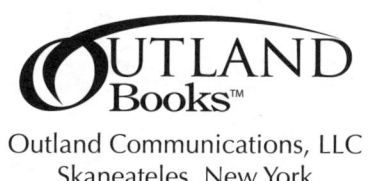

Outland Communications, LLC
Skaneateles, New York

Published by Outland Books
Outland Communications, LLC
P.O. Box 534
4022 Mill Road
Skaneateles, New York 13152

www.outlandbooks.com

ISBN: 1-932820-10-8

Printed in the United States of America

PREFACE

Why the book, *The Best Damn Sex Jokes, Period*? In my experience with both sex and laughter, I've enjoyed each most when they've coincided.

Have fun,
Judy Brown

Web site: www.judybrown.info
Email: judybrowni@usa.net

ACKNOWLEDGEMENTS

I'd like to thank all the comedians who have hilariously mated sex and laughter.

And thanks also to Robert Brown of Outland Books for recognizing that sex (jokes) might sell.

Judy Brown

In a survey, two out of three women said they'd had sex with someone in their office. I can't even get the toner cartridge to go in the copier.

- JAY LENO

I'm not good in bed. Hell, I'm not even good on the couch.

- DREW CAREY

The other night my wife and I decided to spice things up a little. So, we switched positions. She lay on the couch with the remote, and I did the ironing.

- PETER SASSO

They opened up a strip bar in my neighborhood. Big sign out front, "Totally Nude." I thought they meant to get in. So, I'm standing in line...

- MARGARET SMITH

A lot of guys think the larger a woman's breasts are, the less intelligent she is. I think it's the opposite. I think the larger a woman's breasts are, the less intelligent the men become.

                                                    - ANITA WISE

My aunt asked me, "You're a homosexual? Are you seeing a psychiatrist?" "No," I said, "I'm seeing a lieutenant in the army."

                                                    - BOB SMITH

I went to a liberal arts college where a required class was "The History of Dance." But I was annoyed that the professor had so little knowledge of the lap dance. Come on, I'm paying a lot of money to go to school here, know your subject.

                                                    - TONY DEYO

A birth control pill for men, that's fair. It makes more sense to take the bullets out of the gun than to wear a bulletproof vest.

- GREG TRAVIS

(On lesbianism:) One man asked, "Hey, did you get that way because you had some kind of bad sexual experience with a guy?" I'm like, "If that's all it took, the entire female population would be gay, sir."

- SUZANNE WESTENHOEFER

The first time I ever got undressed in front of a woman, it was horrible. She started screaming, and then they kicked me off the bus.

- JAMES LEEMER

Strippers don't like it when you tip them in quarters.

- BIL DWYER

You wanna hear my personal opinion on prostitution? If men knew how to do it, they wouldn't have to pay for it.

> - *ROSEANNE BARR*

My wife insists on turning off the lights when we make love. That doesn't bother me. It's the hiding that seems so cruel.

> - *JONATHAN KATZ*

Sex after children slows down. Every three months now we have sex. Every time I have sex, the next day I pay my quarterly taxes. Unless it's oral sex, then I renew my driver's license.

> - *RAY ROMANO*

A poll shows women think men are sexiest playing football. And they're at their least sexy watching football.

> - *JAY LENO*

(On gays in the military:) Conservatives are worried straight men might become targets of sexual overtures. In other words, men in combat might have to face the same hell that's confronted secretaries and waitresses for generations.

- BEVERLY MICKINS

My mother and I had different attitudes toward sex. She said, "Whatever you do, never sleep with a man until he buys you a house." Well, it worked for her, and I got a swing set out of the deal.

- JUDY BROWN

I think sex is beautiful between the right man and the right woman, but it's difficult to get between the right man and woman.

- WOODY ALLEN

I was performing at a comedy club and when I said I'm a lesbian, a guy in the audience yelled out, "Can I watch?" I said, "Watch me what? Fix my car?"

- SABRINA MATTHEWS

In West Virginia a guy stole $500,000 from a truck parked outside a strip show. Police are questioning a man who's in his third day of a lap dance.

- CRAIG KILBORN

Congress says that half of Americans use the Internet. The other half has sex with real partners.

- JAY LENO

I once made love to a female clown, and she twisted my penis into a poodle.

- DAN WHITNEY

The threesome in sex, when I was single that was sincerely never a fantasy of mine. It was never like, "How could I wake up with two disappointed ladies tomorrow?"

- BOB GOLDTHWAIT

I read in Cosmopolitan that women like to have whipped cream sprayed on their breasts. Unfortunately, my girlfriend has silicone implants. So I use non-dairy topping.

- JEFF SHAW

Never put off for tomorrow who you can put out for tonight.

- JOAN RIVERS

Lots of people think that bisexual means cowardly lesbian.

- SANDRA BERNHARD

Ménage à trois is a French term. It means "Kodak moment."

— GREG RAY

I'd like to open a whorehouse for women so we can get it the way we really want it. Like, we pay our money and guys pretend they like talking to us and they care about our lives, and then they have to hold us real tight and say, "Oooo, you're so thin!" Even if they've never seen us before, they have to say, "Have you lost weight?" Then we have sex, and right before that fabulous moment, they have to shout, "I can't believe how great your shoes match your dress!"

— KAREN HABER

There are more important things than sex. I always thought that music was more important than sex. Then I noticed that if I don't hear a concert for a year-and-a-half, it don't bother me.

— JACKIE MASON

I was watching the game show "Jeopardy." The answer was "French toast." The question was: "What does a very lonely baker do?"

- JOHNNY CARSON

There's now a better Viagra pill that works in a minute instead of an hour. You know a man invented this. It cuts out foreplay completely.

- JAY LENO

Is sex dirty? Only if it's done right.

- WOODY ALLEN

The human race has been set up. Someone, somewhere, is playing a practical joke on us. Apparently, women need to feel loved to have sex. Men need to have sex to feel loved. How do we ever get started?

- BILLY CONNOLLY

One day as I came home early from work, I saw a guy jogging naked. I said to the guy, "Hey buddy, what are you doing that for?" He said, "Because you came home early."

- *RODNEY DANGERFIELD*

I got fired from a job because a woman accused me of sexual harassment. Just because I said, "You look nice today." Through a peephole in the bathroom.

- *KEN FERGUSON*

What's the sexiest four-word sentence in the English language? It's when a Southern woman says, "Hey, y'all, I'm drunk."

- *JEFF FOXWORTHY*

I used to be a virgin, but I gave it up: There was no money in it.

- *MARSHA WARFIELD*

If her lips are on fire and she trembles in your arms, forget her. She's got malaria.

- *JACKIE KANNON*

Love is the answer. But while you're waiting for the answer, sex brings up some pretty good questions.

- *WOODY ALLEN*

They say the best exercise takes place in the bedroom. I believe it, because that's where I get the most resistance.

- *JEFF SHAW*

Exotic dancers at a San Francisco strip club went on strike, and I had to ask myself, what would strippers chant on a picket line? "They said they'd pay us more, but they lied. We want more to be objectified!"

- *NANCY WAITE*

I don't get no respect. A hooker once told me
she had a headache.

> - RODNEY DANGERFIELD

Don't have sex, man. It leads to kissing, and
pretty soon you have to start talking to them.

> - STEVE MARTIN

There's going to be an airline flight from Miami
to Cancun that's nude. I know it sounds like a
good idea, but when the seatbelt sign comes on,
be careful what you fasten.

> - DAVID LETTERMAN

In 1947 the Polaroid camera was invented. The
next day the inventor assured his girlfriend, "I
won't show these to anybody."

> - CONAN O'BRIEN

I urge you all to love yourselves without reservation, and to love each other without restraints. Unless you're into leather. Then, by all means, use restraints.

- MARGARET CHO

My husband says, "Roseanne, don't you think we ought to talk about our sexual problems?" Like I'm gonna turn off *Wheel of Fortune* for that.

- ROSEANNE BARR

I love the lines the men use to get us into bed. "Please, I'll only put it in for a minute." What am I, a microwave?

- BEVERLY MICKINS

I practice safe sex. Some day I'd like to perform it.

- ADAM RICHMOND

Men keep rushing through lovemaking, which is the part I like, the beginning part. Most women are like that. We need time to warm up. Why is this hard for you guys to understand? You are the first people to tell us not to gun a cold engine. You want us to go from zero to sixty in a minute. We're not built like that. We stall.

- ANITA WISE

On a first date recently the woman told me, "I'm bi-sexual." Most men would be thinking, "Woo wee, here comes a three-way!" But this is how I know I'm getting older: I thought, "There's another mouth that won't shut up."

- ERIC WILSON

I tried group sex. Now I have a new problem. I don't know who to thank.

- RODNEY DANGERFIELD

I'm single and dating is hard, and I figured out why. It's those damn romantic comedies. No guy can be this nice, sweet, and understanding. Here's a good example: my ex and I get out of a movie and she turns to me and asks, "Why can't you be more like those guys in the romantic comedies?" So I turned to her and said, "I don't know, why can't you be more like the chicks in pornos?"

- TODD LARSON

The International Olympic Committee has changed their rules, now allowing people who have had sex changes to compete. These people will all be competing in a brand-new event called "What the *hell* is *that*?"

- CONAN O'BRIEN

In 1962 all the expression "safe sex" meant was that you move the bed away from the wall so you wouldn't bang your head.

- DAVID LETTERMAN

I told my kid about the birds and bees. He went out and knocked up a sparrow.

> — RODNEY DANGERFIELD

How many women like to have sex in the morning? How many like to be awake when it happens?

> — MARSHA WARFIELD

Cosmopolitan magazine says that a man reaches his sexual peak at 18, but a woman doesn't reach hers until 35. Of course, we're not talking age, we're talking minutes.

> — TRACI SKENE

Everybody should practice safe sex, because nobody wants to be doing it and put an eye out.

> — EMMY GAY

An 80-year-old woman in Pakistan is pregnant.
You know what she said? "Damn prom."

- *CRAIG KILBORN*

Men and women behave just like our basic
sexual elements. If you watch single men on a
weekend night, they act very much like sperm:
All disorganized, bumping into their friends,
swimming in the wrong direction. "I was first!
Let me through!" "You're on my tail!" "That's
my spot." They're like the Three Billion Stooges.
But the egg is very cool, "Well, who's it going to
be? I can divide. I can wait a month. I'm not
swimming anywhere."

- *JERRY SEINFELD*

I was insecure about sex. I've grown more secure.
I used to use the amateur phylactics, and I only
use the prophylactics now.

- *STEVE MARTIN*

Did you hear about those two strangers who were arrested for having sex in first class on American Airlines? You know who I feel sorry for? The guy in the middle seat.

- JAY LENO

You're born a heterosexual. It's not a choice. Who would choose this? The guilt, the shame... and do you think I'm happy having to hire a decorator?

- GARRY SHANDLING

I said to my husband, "Why don't you call out my name when we're making love?" He said, "I don't want to wake you up."

- JOAN RIVERS

Lead us not into temptation. Just tell us where it is, we'll find it.

- SAM LEVENSON

My parents are in their late sixties and they still have sex. Because they want grandchildren.

- WENDY LIEBMAN

Men are so hung up on penis size. As if the sexiest thing a woman could say in bed is "ouch."

- MIMI GONZALEZ

You get to a certain age, you have a natural sex change. You change from sex to food. You get horny when you see a chocolate chip cookie, and think how much better that would be, and a lot less work.

- MICHELE BALAN

I tried phone sex once, I did. I'll be honest with you. I got my penis stuck in the 9.

- KEVIN MEANEY

How can you have sex without emotional attachment? Use an attachment.

- CARRIE SNOW

According to Men's Health magazine, the average man has had sex in a car fifteen times. That's something to keep in mind next time you're looking for a used car.

- JAY LENO

Women might be able to fake orgasms. But men can fake whole relationships.

- JIMMY SHUBERT

I once dated a waitress. In the middle of sex she'd say, "How is everything? Is everything okay over here?"

- DAVID CORRADO

It's okay to laugh in the bedroom so long as you don't point.

- WILL DURST

When I was growing up you couldn't blow the horn and the girl comes running out. You had to go to the door. Knock on the door. Tell the parents where you are taking their daughter, what time you're gonna have her home. The parents would always come to the door with a dog behind them the size of a horse. The dog starts sniffing your crotch. Now the dog is raising you off the ground. Pretty soon you want to say, "The heck with your daughter, how much do you want for the dog?"

- TOM DREESEN

I married an older man. Foreplay took a little longer, but at least his hand shook.

- JENNY JONES

I believe that sex is a beautiful thing between two people. Between five, it's fantastic.

- *WOODY ALLEN*

I love pizza better than sex. Of course, that's only because I can get pizza.

- *DOUG GRAHAM*

When I was 17 years old, I was going out with a 59-year-old man. Sexually we got along great because the things he couldn't do anymore were the things I didn't know about.

- *CAROL HENRY*

In Texas there's a combination auto repair shop and whorehouse. Don't go there. They always charge you more than the estimate.

- *DAVID LETTERMAN*

A judge declared a mistrial in a pornography case when a male juror went to sleep while they were showing the film. Come on, what guy ever watches a whole porno film?

- JAY LENO

I don't think I'm good in bed. My husband never said anything, but after we made love he'd take a piece of chalk and outline my body.

- JOAN RIVERS

I went to a meeting for premature ejaculators. I left early.

- RED BUTTONS

Casual sex is the best, because you don't have to wear a tie.

- JOHN MENDOZA

Senator Rick Santorum of Pennsylvania compared homosexuality to bigamy, adultery and polygamy. He's tried them all and found them similar. He thinks the only thing a man should put in his mouth is his foot.

- JAY LENO

Sixty percent of women masturbate. The other forty percent expect you to believe it takes that long to take a bath.

- RICHARD JENI

One company has installed a third restroom for a transsexual employee. The employee leaves the toilet seat halfway up.

- CRAIG KILBORN

Hookers don't like to snuggle.

- ZACH GALIFINIAKIS

I support whatever your sexual preference as long as you're committed. I myself can't believe eventually I will have to marry someone the same sex as my mother.

- GARRY SHANDLING

My girlfriend was complaining about my stamina in the old sackeroony, so I popped six Viagras and drank a case of Red Bull. Her funeral is Tuesday.

- HARLAND WILLIAMS

I don't even consider myself bisexual. I just think of myself as a "people person."

- MICHAEL DANE

Ladies, sexually, if your man won't do it, his best friend will.

- LEWIS RAMEY

Playboy was looking for women to star in a Girls of Starbucks pictorial. Ideally, they were looking for venti girls with grande breasts.

- TINA FEY

I've been thinking about S&M lately. Because if the guy ties you up, at least you know he wants you there for a while. It's a commitment.

- JANET ROSEN

Scientists now believe that the primary biological function of breasts is to make males stupid.

- DAVE BARRY

I once made love for an hour and five minutes. It was on the day they push the clock ahead.

- GARRY SHANDLING

Women say they have sexual thoughts too. They have no idea. It's the difference between shooting a bullet and throwing it. If they knew what we were really thinking, they'd never stop slapping us.

- LARRY MILLER

They say men get sexier as they get older. No, sexy men get sexier as they get older, the rest of us get red sports cars.

- JEFF SHAW

I'm taking an art class and the nude model just quit. Because I like to finger-paint.

- WENDY LIEBMAN

I'm smart. This year I'm doing all my Christmas shopping on the Internet. I'm getting everybody porn.

- JAY LENO

Every politician we have, liberal or conservative, who gets caught drinking or chasing women is thrown out of office. It's backwards. It's more dangerous to have a clean-living President with his finger on the button. He thinks he's going right to heaven. You want to feel safe with a leader? Give me a guy who fights in bars and cheats on his wife. This is a man who wants to put off Judgment Day as long as possible.

- LARRY MILLER

I'm getting an abortion. I don't need one, but I feel that as an American I should exercise that right before it gets taken away.

- BETSY SALKIND

I don't need Viagra, I need a pill to help me talk afterwards.

- GARRY SHANDLING

My Web site ends in dot org dot gasm.

- DAVID SPADE

I was such an ugly kid, they made me the poster boy for birth control.

- RODNEY DANGERFIELD

Engaged women have sex 2.9 times a week. And the .9 is really frustrating.

- JAY LENO

If you're looking for a way to piss your mother off, here's what I suggest. Next time you're driving with your mother, stop in front of the local strip joint. Put the car in park and say, "I'll be right back. I just have to run in and pick up my check."

- JUDY GOLD

I had a woman up in my apartment the other night. She gave me the classic line all women give guys on the first date, "Steve, if we do anything tonight we won't be friends." I said, "Hell, I'll find new friends."

– STEVE SMITH

Now that we can clone humans they've removed the one pleasurable thing about having a child.

– DAVID LETTERMAN

A study shows that the more female friends a man has, the less likely he is to have a heart attack, unless his wife catches him with them.

– JAY LENO

What do atheists scream when they cum?

- BILL HICKS

I don't worry too much about sex education in the schools. If the kids learn it like they do everything else, they won't know how.

- MILTON BERLE

Is it bad when you refer to all porno magazines as "dates"?

- PATTON OSWALT

I was making love to this girl and she started crying. I said, "Are you going to hate yourself in the morning?" She said, "No, I hate myself now."

- RODNEY DANGERFIELD

If curling is an Olympic sport, then oral sex is adultery. For that matter, oral sex should be an Olympic sport. I mean, it's harder to do than curling. And, frankly, if you're good at it, you should get a medal.

- LEWIS BLACK

As soon as it's warm I plan to go spelunking with fifty million albino epileptics with tails, just to see how sperm feels.

- BRIAN BEATTY

On the reproductive front, researchers say the number one cause of pregnancy is sex. The number two cause is sex ten minutes later.

- KEVIN NEALON

When porn stars get married, do the guests get to attend the honeymoon?

- JASON LOVE

Animals mate each season. The male picks his female. And then after that season, he's free to pick someone else. How cool is that?

- ROB BITTER

Scientists have now cloned a monkey, and the guys who cloned the sheep are saying, "Who'd want to have sex with a monkey?"

- JAY LENO

You moon the wrong person at an office party and suddenly you're not "professional" any more.

- JEFF FOXWORTHY

I'll tell you what a career is. It's just something you have so you can screw a better class of people.

- TRACY SMITH

I read that when rabbits are having sex, the male rabbit screams, rolls over on his side, and faints. That's reassuring. Because now when I'm driving my car and see a rabbit on the side of the road, I know he's not dead, he just had a date.

- CATHY LADMAN

The guys at strip clubs put a dollar in the stripper's g-string, sit back down. Put a dollar in, sit down. Two in the morning, they're drunk and say to their friends, "Dude, I'm coming back tomorrow. I think she likes me." Sure she likes you, the way a landlord likes you on the first of the month.

- MONIQUE MARVEZ

Sexual harassment at work, is it a problem for the self-employed?

- VICTORIA WOOD

I know I'm not sexy. In high school I was voted Most Likely to Masturbate. They say love thy neighbor as thyself. What am I supposed to do, jerk him off, too?

- RODNEY DANGERFIELD

I blame my mother for my poor sex life. All she told me was, "The man goes on top, and the woman underneath." For three years my husband and I slept in bunk beds.

- JOAN RIVERS

I'm bisexual. Whenever I want sex I can buy it.

- ERIC IDLE

I still remember my prom. I remember pinning the corsage on my prom date, and then she deflated.

- DAVID LETTERMAN

Gay men in drag think it's glamorous being a woman, that it's all about the dress and make-up. Hey buddy, if you really want to impersonate a woman shove a tampon up your wazoo every month, give birth, and take a cut in pay.

- MICHELE BALAN

Men reach their sexual peak at 18. Women reach their sexual peak at 35. Do you get the feeling God is into practical jokes? We're reaching our sexual peak right around the same time they're discovering they have a favorite chair.

- RITA RUDNER

As part of a mass wedding ceremony in Thailand, "Guy," a chicken, married "Guk," a rooster. And, for the record, on their wedding night, the chicken came first.

- JIMMY FALLON

New York hotels are providing condoms in every room. And the nicer hotels will even leave a mint on your penis.

- CONAN O'BRIEN

Last week I told my wife, "If you would learn to cook, I could fire the chef." She said, "If you could learn to make love, I could fire the chauffeur."

- RODNEY DANGERFIELD

Doctors in India have performed the first penis transplant. It's a great excuse for cheating. "It wasn't even mine. The guy who used to have it was a pig."

- JAY LENO

Hooters Air is off the ground. In the event of a water landing, there'll be a wet T-shirt contest.

- CRAIG KILBORN

He said, "I love you terribly." She said, "You certainly do."

- HENNY YOUNGMAN

Girls who put out are tramps. Girls who don't are ladies. This is, however, a rather archaic usage of the word. Should one of you boys happen upon a girl who doesn't put out, do not jump to the conclusion that you have found a lady. What you have probably found is a lesbian.

- FRAN LEBOWITZ

In a test program, 40 drugstores in Washington state will be dispensing morning-after birth control pills without prescriptions. In fact, men can buy them in special gift pacts with cards that say, "Thanks, maybe I'll call you sometime."

- JAY LENO

Oh yes, I've tried my hand at sex.

- EMO PHILIPS

My mom always said, "Men are like linoleum floors. You lay them right, and you can walk on them for thirty years."

- BRETT BUTLER

My father raised me by the good book. Although, to tell the truth, I've never been able to locate that verse about the electric nipple clamp.

- EMO PHILIPS

I'm in kind of a sexual dry spell. For the past few years, I've only had sex in the months that end in "arch."

- DOUG BENSON

It's hard for me to get used to these changing times. I can remember when the air was clean and sex was dirty.

- GEORGE BURNS

When we got married, I told my wife I like sex twice a day. She said, "Me too." Now we never see each other.

- RODNEY DANGERFIELD

I learn so much from my teenage daughter. We're in the car, listening to the radio and she says, "Yeah, that Foxy Brown, she's got an ill nana. You know what an ill nana is?" A sick grandma? No, in Ebonics ill and sick and mad are all good, and a nana is a vagina. "Oh," I said to my daughter, "I used to have an ill nana, but then I had you."

- CORY KAHANE

An Australian gay guy disgusted with the men in the U.S.A.: "I'm going back to my Sydney!"

- HENNY YOUNGMAN

Sex after a fight is often the best there is, which is why you're never allowed in the locker room right after a prizefight.

- JAY LENO

I think the size of breast implants is just crazy. To me it looks like they come in three sizes: Large, Extra Large and Holy Smoke! But I guess there are some advantages to having breasts that big. On a picnic you basically have your own table and it seats six.

- JENNIFER POST

There are 25,000 sex phone lines for men in the U.S. but only three for women. Apparently, when we want somebody to talk dirty and nasty to us we just go to work.

- FELICIA MICHAELS

My uncle's so lazy he married a girl who was already pregnant.

- RODNEY DANGERFIELD

I once saw my grandparents have sex, and that's why I don't eat raisins.

- ZACH GALIFINIAKIS

Tom Green in Utah has five wives. One is the head wife, and I'm not going to comment on that. That's her title. The penalty for five wives is five mothers-in-law.

- JAY LENO

Swingers cheat on each other together.

- JASON LOVE

The only way to really have safe sex is to abstain. From drinking.

- WENDY LIEBMAN

Phone sex, my worst fantasy. "You're thinking dirty thoughts?" "Yeah." "Okay, your mother wants to talk to you."

- ROBERT SCHIMMEL

I happen to like old-school '70s porn because I like the natural body. The women in this new porn, their boobs are just so weird and high and far out, they look like those goldfish with the puffy eyes.

- MARGARET CHO

Men and women just look at life completely different. Women are playing chess, we plan relationships ten moves ahead. Meanwhile, the guy is playing checkers, thinking just one move ahead: "Jump me!"

- MARGOT BLACK

I've done a little survey, guys, and size does matter. But not as much as smell.

- DANIEL LIEBERT

Humans are the only animal who can have sex over the phone.

- DAVID LETTERMAN

Those S&M people are bossy.

- MARGARET CHO

According to the *British Journal of Psychiatry*, men cope with infidelity with denial. That's not true! That's a lie! I refuse to believe that!

- JAY LENO

I could never be comfortable at an orgy. I'd always think there would be someone making rabbit ears behind my back.

- DIANE NICHOLS

You wake up one day and say, "You know what, I don't think I ever need to sleep or have sex again." Congratulations, you're ready to have children.

- RAY ROMANO

Why does a guy say "I'm seeing her" when he really means "I'm touching her?"

- JASON LOVE

Oh, she's a wild girl. Her idea of safe sex is making sure the car doors are locked.

- RODNEY DANGERFIELD

I quit a job once because of sexual harassment. There was nowhere near enough of it going on to keep me around. I've got needs.

- MEL FINE

Men love oral sex because it combines the two activities that the average guy never gets tired of: 1) Sex, and 2) Not moving at all. If the Superbowl was on I could die right now.

- RICHARD JENI

In Italy an 85-year-old man and a 75-year-old woman were arrested for having sex in a parked car, and the left-turn signal was on the whole time.

- JAY LENO

It's so long since I've had sex, I've forgotten who gets tied up.

- JOAN RIVERS

Pornography confuses me. I don't understand how every month so many women with so few teeth get their pictures in *Hustler* magazine's Beaver Hunt.

- BRIAN BEATTY

Viagra is the work of the devil. Now we girls can look forward to having sex with really old guys, for a really long time.

- LEMAIRE

My girlfriend is taking acting lessons, so she can fake it better. And I'm nervous, because next week is the final project and the entire class is coming over to watch.

- CRAIG SHARF

When my daughter was six she started asking embarrassing questions. Luckily, we had gotten her two hamsters, and about a week later she had four hamsters. So I explained that when a boy hamster and a girl hamster love each other, and make a commitment, they can have baby hamsters. A week after that she had 20 hamsters, so I had to tell her about incest.

- JONATHAN KATZ

Sex at the age of eighty-four is a wonderful experience. Especially the one in the winter.

- MILTON BERLE

In a poll, 76% of men said they wouldn't get serious about a woman who slept with them on the first date. They would, however, be very serious about getting a second date.

- JAY LENO

I hate my voice because I don't think it's sexy. I got an obscene phone call, and I actually felt guilty because I thought I turned the guy off.

- CATHY LADMAN

A recent study said that, because of their exposure to emissions, sperm counts tend to be lower in truck drivers and toll collectors. I think I speak for all of us when I say, "Whew."

- MARK STILES

I haven't had sex in so long I'm starting to have wet dreams about masturbating.

- ADAM RICHMOND

My husband says I don't understand pornography because I'm always fast-forwarding to the story.

- ALICIA BRANDT

I am so unprejudiced that I never notice a person's race or sexual orientation until it is much, much too late.

- STRANGE DE JIM

Every porno movie should be called "Stuff That Never Happens to You."

- RICHARD JENI

Which came first, the chicken or the egg? It was neither. Being a typical male, the rooster came first.

- TONY INVERGO

In Germany a man got his manhood caught in his vacuum cleaner. He told the doctors the relationship was purely sexual. He didn't want any attachments.

- *JAY LENO*

My sister and brother-in-law say they're practicing nudists. Now I ask you, how do you practice naked? Either you is, or you ain't. Perhaps they need the book, "Naked for Dummies." I'll get them the hard copy.

- *KATHIE DICE*

Phone sex, I got an ear infection.

- *RICHARD LEWIS*

They say that baseball is the national pastime, but I think it's looking at women's rear ends.

- *JASON LOVE*

I used to have a girlfriend who would blow me when I drove. It wasn't every time I drove, but every time I drove into a tree.

— ADAM RICHMOND

Some women can't say the word "lesbian," even when their mouth is full of one.

— KATE CLINTON

Monogamous sex is what one partner in every relationship wants it to be.

— STRANGE DE JIM

A woman won't dump a man until she's found someone to replace him. In a woman's mind, if you cheat on her it's because you're a jerk. But if she cheats on you, it's because you're a jerk.

— JEFF SHAW

I was at a fancy restaurant. They had a waiter for everything. The butter waiter came over and gave us butter, the water waiter came over and gave us water, the head waiter came over — oh, it was so fancy.

- GEORGE MILLER

I tell ya, I got no sex life. My dog watched me in the bedroom, to learn how to beg. He also taught my wife how to roll over and play dead.

- RODNEY DANGERFIELD

This gay wedding craze is starting to spread around the country. Today, a guy in Utah married five other guys.

- JAY LENO

Dr. Ruth says women should tell our lovers how to make love to us. My boyfriend goes nuts if I tell him how to drive.

- PAM STONE

Men are always calling me a strong woman. I hate when I hear that because it only means one thing: I have to be on top all night long.

- JENNIFER FAIRBANKS

I practice safe sex. I use an airbag. It's a little startling at first when it flies out. Then the woman realizes it's safer than being thrown clear.

- GARRY SHANDLING

I read books that say if you want to keep sex hot, you tell the person what you want. How do you tell them you want somebody else?

- ELAYNE BOOSLER

A Texas man was arrested for masturbating in public. He doesn't want a lawyer. He says he can get himself off.

- CONAN O'BRIEN

Dr. Joyce brothers said that "Men have a sexual thought every other minute." Who are these guys, and why do they wait so long?"

- TOM DREESEN

I saw a blind man rent a porno video. He must really like bad music.

- MARK GROSS

The fad now is wearing T-shirts with your area code. You can tell a lot about people. For instance, if a woman has a 900 number.

- JAY LENO

I wonder, is pain always sexual for S&M people? If they're walking down the street, and they stub their toe, do they go, "Ow! I'm so horny."

– SUZANNE WESTENHOEFER

I had to learn about sex from porno movies. That doesn't work. Learning sex from porno, that's like learning how to drive by watching the Indianapolis 500.

– NORMAN K.

The Chinese government is banning the TV show "Friends" because it has too much sex on it. You wouldn't want to send a country with nine billion people down the wrong road.

– CRAIG KILBORN

I'm writing a new sitcom for HBO, "Sex in the Suburbs." It's about a five-minute show.

– BETH DAVIDOFF

Sex at age 90 is like trying to shoot pool with a rope. I'm at the age now where just putting my cigar in its holder is a thrill.

- GEORGE BURNS

Men love to watch two women make love. I wonder, does this turn them on, or are they just trying to figure out how to do it right?

- JOY BEHAR

A woman in Great Britain is suing because her kid's Incredible Hulk doll had a two-inch penis. And that's before he got angry.

- JAY LENO

With my wife, I gave up. The other night, I told her, "You win, you're the boss. When it comes to sex, it'll be in your hands." She said, "You're wrong, it'll be in your hands."

- RODNEY DANGERFIELD

Did you ever have a sex cramp in your leg? My leg gets going and my dog is looking at me like, "That's the way, Bobby. That's what we call doggie style."

- BOBBY COLLINS

I was a virgin until I was 20. And then again, until I was 23.

- CARRIE SNOW

Here's an odd fact: The first nudist organization in America was established on this date in 1929. Boy, that's one group you don't want to see have a reunion, huh?

- JAY LENO

Sex is not the answer. Sex is the question. "Yes" is the answer.

- SWAMI X

I'm a quadrasexual. That means I'll do anything with anyone for a quarter.

- ED BLUESTONE

My impression of an atheist making love: "Ohhh, nobody!"

- STAN SCHACTER

A man goes to a barbershop and asks, "How many ahead of me?" "Five." The man leaves. He comes back tomorrow and asks, "How many ahead of me." "Four." The man leaves. He comes back the next day and asks, "How many ahead of me?" "Six." The man leaves, and the barber says to another, "Follow that guy!" The man comes back and says, "He goes to your house."

- HENNY YOUNGMAN

A new machine for passenger screening at airports sees right through clothing. Listen, if it keeps the screeners awake...

- CONAN O'BRIEN

My last boyfriend liked to talk a lot during sex. He said it was because it turned him on, but I think he had ulterior motives because he always said he same thing, "Wake up, wake up, wake up!"

- CHRISTINE O'ROURKE

Having sex is like playing bridge. If you don't have a good partner, you'd better have a good hand.

- WOODY ALLEN

Making love to a woman is like buying real estate: Location, location, location.

- CAROL LEIFER

There's a type of food that makes women give up oral sex: wedding cake.

- BILL MAHER

There's a new medical crisis. Doctors are reporting that many men are having allergic reactions to latex condoms. They say they cause severe swelling. So what's the problem?

- JAY LENO

Happiness is watching the TV at your girlfriend's house during a power failure.

- BOB HOPE

A lot of stuff in school you don't appreciate until you get to be older. Little things, like being spanked every day by a middle-aged woman. Stuff you'd pay good money for later in life.

- EMO PHILIPS

I can't express my sexual needs, except to strangers over the phone. Then I can go for hours, even through that loud whistle.

- *GARRY SHANDLING*

My man won't open my door or pull out my chair. But the minute we're alone, he wants to open my legs and pull down my undies.

- *LAURIE MCDERMOTT*

It's not true that rubbing a toad will give you warts. However, it will give the toad a hard-on.

- *GEORGE CARLIN*

Men in power always seem to get involved in sex scandals, but women don't even have a word for male bimbo. Except maybe, "Senator."

- *ELAYNE BOOSLER*

Animal rights activists are protesting the running of the bulls in Pamplona. Naked women are going to run through the streets in protest. Yeah, that'll keep the guys away. You don't want to get gored by a 36-D cup.

- JAY LENO

If sex is such a natural phenomenon, how come there are so many books on how to do it?

- BETTE MIDLER

You know what I say about edible panties? I say if you're drunk enough, and your teeth are sharp enough, every panty is edible.

- BRIAN MCKIM

I asked my wife to try anal sex. She said, "Sure. You first."

- ROBERT SCHIMMEL

My take on marriage is this: Why buy the butcher when you can get the sausage for free?

- *JEN KERWIN*

The other night in bed my wife was saying sexy things. I looked up, and she was on the phone.

- *RODNEY DANGERFIELD*

The problem is that God gives men a brain and a penis, and only enough blood to run one at a time.

- *ROBIN WILLIAMS*

Women reading *Vogue* magazine about the latest fashions to come off the Paris runway is the same as you men looking at naked women in *Playboy*. We're both looking at places we're never going to be.

- *ANDI RHOADS*

This morning I found a spider in my bed, and I thought, "Gee, I must have been drunk."

- FRED WOLF

Utah is eliminating the porn czar, the guy who had to look at all the porn. I feel sorry for the next guy to get his desk.

- JAY LENO

Twelve hundred women a year are getting pregnant at Fort Polk. That's why they call it Fort Polk. And that's why they call them drill sergeants.

- BILL MAHER

After making love I said to my girl, "Was it good for you, too?" And she said, "I don't think that was good for anybody."

- GARRY SHANDLING

My wife was afraid of the dark. Then she saw me naked. Now she's afraid of the light.

- RODNEY DANGERFIELD

I'm scared of sex now. You have to be. You can get something terminal, like a kid.

- WENDY LIEBMAN

My last girlfriend was pretty wild in bed. She used to cover me from head to toe with oil, and then set me on fire.

- DAVID CORRADO

My friends hired a male stripper for my birthday present. This guy starts throwing his clothes off, and asks me, "What are you thinking, baby?" I'm thinking I've been married too long, because I said, "You're going to pick up after yourself, aren't you?"

- MARY PFEIFFER

I spent the night at Neverland Ranch. We had milk and cookies and got into our pajamas. It was all perfectly innocent. But the odd thing was: only one pair of pajamas. And then in the morning I helped Michael Jackson bleach his penis.

- CHRIS ELLIOT

A study says taking birth control pills makes a woman's voice more pleasant. Of course. "Yes" is always more pleasant than "no."

- JAY LENO

A woman was taking a shower. There is a knock on the door. "Who is it?" "Blind man." The woman opens the door, naked. "Where do you want these blinds, lady?"

- HENNY YOUNGMAN

Freud accused women of having penis envy. I have no reason to be jealous of a penis. At least when I get out of the ocean, all my bodily parts are still the same size.

- SHEILA WENZ

Australian scientists say contraception is thousands of years old, and the first contraceptive was the jaw bone from a yak. The woman would hit the guy over the head with it.

- JAY LENO

NASA announced today that they will begin researching sex in space. They're already printing bumper stickers that say, "If this shuttle's a rockin', don't come a dockin'."

- CONAN O'BRIEN

I don't respect prostitutes. I think they've sold out.

- CRAIG SHARF

This is why there are so many sexual harassment suits today: Guys watch the porno movies and get a warped view of reality. If you watch enough dirty movies you can only come to the conclusion: Hey, women get really horny in the Xerox room! Next thing you know, there's a guy in a real life office with a real life woman, she's at the Xerox machine. He pops up, "Hey honey, I've got a huge boner." "What?" I said, "That machine is out of toner. I'm gonna go back to my office now."

— RICHARD JENI

My orgies are like the Special Olympics. Lots of drooling, but everybody's a winner.

— MATT WEINHOLD

Aren't all parades pretty much gay?

— JASON LOVE

I sent my dog to obedience school and she liked it. Now she wants to get tied up and whipped.

> - ED BLUESTONE

I had sex for five hours once, but four-and-a-half was apologizing.

> - CONAN O'BRIEN

According to a new study, men who drive Porsches are the most likely to have extramarital affairs. Do you know who have the least affairs? Guys who ride the bus.

> - JAY LENO

That's why I'm afraid of marriage. You have to make love to the same person for, like, three hundred years. How do you keep it exciting? Hats?

> - ELAYNE BOOSLER

Sexually, my wife is very responsive. Trouble is, her response is always "No."

- RENO GOODALE

The only time my wife and I had a simultaneous orgasm was when the judge signed the divorce papers.

- WOODY ALLEN

I went out with this one guy, I was very excited about it. He took me out to dinner, he made me laugh, he made me pay. He's like, "Oh, I'm sorry. I forgot my wallet." "Really? I forgot my vagina."

- LISA SUNDSTEDT

I asked a cab driver, "Where can I get some action?" He took me to my house.

- RODNEY DANGERFIELD

A psychic woman claims to be able to tell a man's future by having sex with him. Can't every woman do this? You have sex, and the man falls asleep.

- CRAIG KILBORN

I was with this girl the other night and from the way she was responding to my skillful caresses, you would have sworn that she was conscious, from the top of her head to the tag on her toes.

- EMO PHILIPS

A guy complains of a headache. Another guy says, "Do what I do. I put my head on my wife's bosom, and the headache goes away." The next day, the man says, "Did you do what I told you to?" "Yes, I sure did. By the way, you have a nice house."

- HENNY YOUNGMAN

I just broke up with my girlfriend, because I caught her lying. Under another man.

- DOUG BENSON

Women need a reason to have sex. Men just need a place.

- BILLY CRYSTAL

Into bondage? I am. What I do when I'm in the mood is tie her up, and gag her, and go into the living room and watch football.

- TOM ARNOLD

According to a new survey, women say they feel more comfortable undressing in front of men than they do undressing in front of other women. They say that women are too judgmental, where, of course, men are just grateful.

- JAY LENO

There's a double standard, even today. A man can sleep around and sleep around, and nobody asks any questions. A woman, you make 19 or 20 mistakes, right away you're a tramp.

- JOAN RIVERS

One night I figured I'd let my wife make the first move. She went to Florida.

- RODNEY DANGERFIELD

We should pass a new law: Nobody can get famous just by sleeping with a celebrity, and getting naked in a magazine. You have to make a contribution to society, first. You can still be in *Playboy*, you just have to do something worthwhile beforehand. "I developed a vaccine, and I'd like to show you my breasts." Go ahead, you've earned it.

- ELAYNE BOOSLER

Anyone who calls it "sexual intercourse" can't possibly be interested in actually doing it. You might as well announce you're ready for lunch by proclaiming, "I'd like to do some masticating and enzyme secreting."

- ALLAN SHERMAN

I think women should date younger men. Thirty-five, forty-year-old women are peaking when 18-year-old boys are peaking, and that's who we should be peaking and poking.

- SHEILA KAY

At the L.A. zoo, the zookeeper is having a tough time keeping the animals from getting pregnant. This is true; they have to force feed the female chimps to get them to swallow the birth control pills. Hey, it's a lot easier than trying to get the male chimps to wear a condom.

- JAY LENO

I tell ya, it's lonely at the top when there's no one on the bottom.

- RODNEY DANGERFIELD

My boyfriend had a W tattooed on each cheek. So when he bends over it says, "Wow!"

- MARGARET SMITH

Half of Americans say they've had sex on the job. No wonder foreign workers are trying to sneak into the country.

- JAY LENO

When I was nine, I caught my father cheating with another woman. I was a good kid. I didn't tell. But my friends wondered why my allowance went up to $900 a week.

- BILLY RIBACK

A guy says, "I'm so old that I forgot how old I am." An old woman says, "I'll tell you how old you are. Take off your clothes and bend over." The man does this. The woman says, "You're seventy four." The man says, "How can you tell?" The woman says, "You told me yesterday."

- HENNY YOUNGMAN

According to a group of scientists, a new study claims that teenage lesbians have a higher chance of smoking than straight girls. Another study also reveals that guys who do studies would rather study teenage lesbians than almost anything else in the world.

- JAY LENO

If it wasn't for pickpockets and frisking at airports I'd have no sex life at all.

- RODNEY DANGERFIELD

I never believed in casual sex. I have always tried as hard as I could.

- GARRY SHANDLING

In a survey for *Modern Maturity* magazine, men over 75 said they had sex once a week. Which proves that old guys lie about sex, too.

- IRV GILMAN

The cable TV sex channels don't expand our horizons, don't make us better people, and don't come in clearly enough.

- BILL MAHER

Hooters Air is a low-cost airline that features young women in hot pants and tank tops serving snacks. And, in the event of an emergency, the women can be used as a floatation device.

- TINA FEY

My girlfriend always laughs during sex, no matter what she's reading.

- EMO PHILIPS

Ninety percent of men masturbate. The other ten percent don't have arms.

- RICHARD JENI

Tonight on the news I saw two gay men getting married. That's really incredible when I think about it, two men who want to get married. At most weddings you don't even have one guy.

- JAY LENO

Women are getting this laser surgery to tighten up their vaginas. Men are going on the internet to get a huge penis. Hey, I'm not Nostradamus, but I sense trouble.

- DANIEL LIEBERT

I grew up in a strict Catholic home, and I didn't have Sex Education until I got to college. Man, I didn't know it was that easy to get an A.

- LEAH EVA

My mother is 60, and her whole life she only slept with one guy. She won't tell me who.

- WENDY LIEBMAN

I was on a date, and this girl teased a banana in a suggestive manner and said, "That could be you." I replied, "Well then, I should probably get that dark, soft-spot looked at."

- DERIC HARRINGTON

No matter what she says or does, remember one thing: all women want it. But maybe not with *you*.

- BILL KALMENSON

In the middle of an asthma attack, my sister got an obscene phone call. The guy said, "Did I call you, or did you call me?"

- JOHN MENDOZA

Hackers even shut down some porn sites. People had to have sex the old-fashioned way, over the phone.

- JAY LENO

They say you should always wear a condom, but I've noticed that after about three weeks it starts feeling itchy.

- THE COVERT COMIC

No other character could possibly be as sexually satisfied as the wife of the Energizer Bunny.

- ROB O'REILLY

Those stupid laws that say the person being breast-fed in public has to be a baby.

- NORM MACDONALD

I'm trying to get stress out of my life. I had a massage about a month ago. Have you had one? Did they put the whipped cream on you, too? It's a weird thing the first time getting a massage because you're lying on a table naked, being touched by a stranger. Which is very, very nice. They try and relax you. He played music, which was a little aggravating. The trombone kept hitting me in the head... at least I think it was a trombone.

- ELLEN DEGENERES

The sodomy laws have been overturned, so now we can overturn each other.

- CRAIG KILBORN

People want to take sex education out of the schools. They believe sex education causes promiscuity. Hey, I took algebra. I never do math.

— ELAYNE BOOSLER

When authorities warn you of the sinfulness of sex, there is an important lesson to be learned. Do not have sex with the authorities.

— MATT GROENING

For the first time in Philadelphia, a policeman got a sex change and became a policewoman. When a man becomes a woman, you know what the most painful cut is? Salary.

— JAY LENO

Never tell your wife she's lousy in bed. She'll go out and get a second opinion.

- RODNEY DANGERFIELD

Women who experimented with lesbianism in college but have gone back to men are called "hasbiens."

- JAY LENO

The most precious gift you can give to a man is your virginity. I ought to know, I've given it to at least a dozen men.

- LIVIA SQUIRES

I was thrown out of the Army for contributing to the delinquency of a major.

- STRANGE DE JIM

When you've been married a long time, sex is like a kite that will only fly when you run with it. Sometimes my wife spices up our marriage. Candlelight, massage, incense, its great, but I'm almost embarrassed. "All this for me?" It's like a chef making sauces, and firing up a little weenie.

- DANIEL LIEBERT

For a woman the worst thing about a sperm bank is that sperm is no longer free. Just go into a bar, and a sperm container will try to pick you up.

- TINA GEORGIE

I told my doctor I want a vasectomy. He said with a face like mine, I don't need one.

- RODNEY DANGERFIELD

Strip poker is the only game in which the more you lose, the more you have to show for it.

- HENNY YOUNGMAN

A woman has given birth to the first cloned baby. At least that's what she's telling her husband, who had a vasectomy.

- JAY LENO

This year, I hope to get something different for my birthday: laid.

- RENO GOODALE

An Austrian man is in good spirits after receiving a tongue transplant. His wife is in even better spirits.

- CONAN O'BRIEN

Everyone in my family asks me, "When are you getting married?" Which means, "We know you're doing it, and we're tired of feeding you."

- MONIQUE MARVEZ

Some men think that they can convert gay women, make them straight. I couldn't do that. I could make a straight woman gay, though.

- JEFF STILSON

A group of students at Harvard University caused controversy by sculpting a nine-foot penis out of ice on campus. The sculpture had to be taken down after 10 Wellesley girls got their tongues stuck to it.

- TINA FEY

You know you've been married for a long time when you're about to engage in some hot, passionate love-making and just as you look lovingly into your wife's eyes, she tells you that she hasn't had a shower in two days. And you still want to get it on.

- DON MCLYSAGHT

In bed my wife sprawls out all over the mattress.
I said, "I'm tired of only having two inches in this
bed." She said "Now you know how I feel."

- PETER SASSO

My ex-wife was multi-orgasmic. Married nine
years, two orgasms. And I wasn't there for either
of them; some guys at work told me about it.

- KEN FERGUSON

Playboy magazine's Miss November of 1992
has come out of the closet and admits she's a
lesbian. She says she realized she was a lesbian
at the Playboy Mansion, right after she saw Hugh
Hefner naked.

- JAY LENO

Everybody lies about sex. People lie during sex.
If it weren't for lies, there'd be no sex.

- JERRY SEINFELD

Have you ever faked orgasm while masturbating?

- JANICE HEISS

They say you can't tell guys are gay just by looking. But if two guys are kissing, you can figure at least one of them is gay.

- BILL BRAUDIS

The Bible contains six admonishments to homosexuals, and 362 to heterosexuals. This doesn't mean God doesn't love heterosexuals; it's just that they need more supervision.

- LYNN LAVNER

New York City hotels have free condoms in the rooms. All these years I've been using the free shower cap.

- DAVID LETTERMAN

The best contraceptive for old people is nudity.

- PHYLLIS DILLER

I was once a stripper. I took off my jewelry and said, "According to Jewish law, I am now naked."

- CHARISSE SAVARIN

People always brag about their sex lives. Why shouldn't you brag about your masturbating life? "Gather around boys, I've got a story for you. I got home Tuesday and I'm alone. I know, I didn't think anything was going to happen either. The next thing you know, I shut the lights, boom! I'm all over myself like a cheap suit. Upstairs, downstairs, I am the best I've ever had."

- RICHARD JENI

I watched zebras mate on the Discovery Channel to see if a zebra erection looks like a barber pole.

- RICHARD LEWIS

The other night I was making love to my wife, and she said, "Deeper, deeper." So I started quoting Nietsche to her.

- DENNIS MILLER

Today a post office was shut down, but a vibrating box turned out to contain a vibrator. Police suspect a single woman acting alone.

- CRAIG KILBORN

A study shows that monogamous couples live longer. And cheaters who don't get caught live longer than cheaters who do get caught.

- JAY LENO

Here's my recipe for inexpensive phone sex. Call for the time of day and start shouting, "All right, slut, say it again — and add ten seconds!"

- JIM SAMUELS

I was dating a control freak. He insisted that he take the birth control pills.

- WENDY LEIBMAN

Environmentalists announced that two dams on a river in Maine are to be torn down in an effort to encourage salmon to return to the river to spawn. Also encouraging salmon to spawn: salmon porn.

- JIMMY FALLON

I hate phone solicitors. I'd rather get an obscene call; at least they work for themselves.

- MARGARET SMITH

I've had more women than most people have noses.

- STEVE MARTIN

I'm Catholic. My mother and I were unpacking and she found my diaphragm. I had to tell her it was a bathing cap for my cat.

- LIZZ WINSTEAD

A new study says sex before a marathon is a good thing. Now men can legitimately say, "Sorry, babe, gotta run."

- JAY LENO

My therapist always says that you should be friends with someone before you sleep with them. But the truth of the matter is, once you get to know someone, who the hell wants to have sex with them?

- JUDY CARTER

I've decided to get a tattoo of parsley on my inner thigh, because presentation is everything.

- GRACE WHITE

I went to a strip club, totally nude. Sure, my testicles stuck to the chair...

- BIL DWYER

It's the 50th anniversary of *Playboy* magazine. Did you realize you can go back in the archives and find the exact Playmate your grandfather was imagining when he created your dad?

- CRAIG KILBORN

Japanese women are refusing to take birth control pills, opting to leave contraception up to men. Do you know what they call women who leave birth control up to men? Mothers.

- JENNIFER VALLY

Men perform oral sex like they drive. When they get lost they refuse to ask for directions.

- CATHERINE FRANCO

"Crimes of passion." That phrase drives me crazy. A man murdering his girlfriend is not a crime of passion. Premature ejaculation: that's a crime of passion.

- HELLURA LYLE

Teenage pregnancy is on the rise. Kids are getting pregnant younger and younger these days. It's even a problem in some middle schools. But I think I have a solution. You take the kids to one of those big IMAX theaters and you show them "Debbie Does Dallas." If I'd seen a seven-story vagina when I was in middle school, I'm pretty sure I'd still be a virgin today.

- TONY DEYO

I'm in favor of gay marriage. Then at least both people are excited about planning the wedding.

- JAY LENO

Forty-six percent of women surveyed answered "Yes" when asked if they ever faked an orgasm. Actually they said, "Yes, yes! Oh God, yes!"

- WAYNE COTTER

When you get a good look at the guy in a dirty movie you go, "Ah ha! No wonder this isn't happening to me. This guy has a member bigger than some of your major household appliances." Whereas you could have sex with a Cheerio without breaking it.

- RICHARD JENI

A group is organizing the first airline flights for nudists. I don't even like the guy in the next seat touching me with his elbow. And Palm Springs is building the first nudist bridge. How'd you like to be the toll taker? "Hey, this quarter's warm!"

- JAY LENO

Japanese women inherit their breasts from their fathers.

- TAMAYO OTSUKI

Safe sex is very important. That's why I'm never doing it on plywood scaffolding again.

- JENNY JONES

They say that lesbians hate men. Why would a lesbian hate a man? They don't have to fuck them.

- ROSEANNE BARR

I've had a lot of nice compliments after making love. Stuff like, "I wanted to moan, but I didn't have time."

- ED BLUESTONE

If you think your sex life might need a little spicing up, and you should find yourself, say, in a sex shop, let me give you some advice: Don't buy the chocolate body frosting. It takes 60 licks per square centimeter to get it off, and that stuff is filling. Basically, you're not going to get much out of it, unless you're the kind of person who only feels sexy after a big Thanksgiving dinner.

- LISA SCHROEER

In college I experimented with heterosexuality: I slept with a straight guy. I was really drunk.

- BOB SMITH

Magnum condoms are a marketing gimmick, because what guy is going admit he doesn't require them? "No thanks. They're so big on me, I need to use a twist tie."

- ROBERT SCHIMMEL

In Berlin a laundromat was raided because it was a front for a brothel. You know what tipped police off? Men doing laundry.

- JAY LENO

A new survey reveals that women would rather give up sex than give up the remote for the TV. Men, on the other hand, would be willing to have sex *with* the remote for the TV.

- CONAN O'BRIEN

The Web brings people together because no matter what kind of a twisted sexual mutant you happen to be, you've got millions of pals out there. Type in, "Find people who have sex with goats that are on fire," and the computer will say, "Specify type of goat."

- RICHARD JENI

I had a cat once. That was the roughest night of sex I ever had.

— MATT VANCE

I wanted my last girlfriend to get into role-playing in bed. But she would always say, "Just put the dice away."

— MYQ KAPLAN

A new study says that having sex decreases your chances of getting a cold. The more sex you have, the less you'll have a cold. Just wait until guys get hold of this. A woman sneezes and he'll be saying, "Hey, I got something for that."

— JAY LENO

I used to pose nude for painters. House painters.

— CINDY HEIDEL

I was once asked to play Strip Poker, but I'm more comfortable with Strip Solitaire.

- ROB O'REILLY

Last time I tried to make love to my wife, nothing was happening, so I said to her, "What's the matter, you can't think of anybody either?"

- RODNEY DANGERFIELD

There's a product called Mr. Big Cream. Just rub it on your dick and it gets bigger. Well, if it worked, then wouldn't your hands get bigger, too?

- ROBERT SCHIMMEL

Don't you hate it when you date someone and they say, "I love you, but I'm not *in* love with you"? You just want to go, "I want you, but not inside me."

- FELICIA MICHAELS

One of my friends was getting married, and they tell me I have to chip in for a male stripper. Are you out of your damn mind? I ain't paying for no naked-ass man. Women don't have to pay to see that. We spend most of our time trying *not* to see that.

- WANDA SYKES

I never will forget my granny… One day she's sitting out on the porch and I said, "Granny, how old does a woman get before she don't want no more boyfriends?" She was around 106 then. She said, "I don't know, honey, you'll have to ask somebody older than me."

- MOMS MABLEY

It's too much trouble to get laid. Because you have to go out with a guy, and go to dinner with him, and listen to him talk about his opinions. And I don't have that kind of time.

- KATHY GRIFFIN

I bet the Marquis de Sade would have liked the Three Stooges.

- DAVID CORRADO

I'm afraid to give instructions in bed because I'm afraid I'll get carried away. "Okay, pull my hair, and touch me right there. No, to the left. Now go outside and move my car so I won't get a ticket. Yeah, that's it."

- LAURA KIGHTLINGER

Larry Flynt is now spokesman for organ donation. How novel of him to be hocking his own body parts for a change.

- BETSY SALKIND

I heard that having a mirror over your bed was supposed to be romantic. A week later I caught somebody shoplifting in my apartment.

- ELAYNE BOOSLER

I see a woman in a bar, and she's drinking my favorite drink: A lot. So I pick her up, and we go to my place and do it doggie style. It wasn't my idea. That's just the position in which she passed out.

- DAVE ATTELL

My personal history: I started out as a sperm. Good swimmer. Liked eggs. Nine months, mom kicks me out of my first home. Since then, I've been living on the outside and looking for similar accommodations. I find them occasionally, but I make a mess and have to leave.

- BASIL WHITE

I wear two condoms all the time. Then when I make love, I take one off, and I feel like a wild man.

- DENNIS MILLER

How did sex come to be thought of as dirty in the first place? God must have been a Republican.

- WILL DURST

When did cuddling go out of style? When did that become a bad thing? Last night I was making love with a prostitute and she gets up to walk out the door, the car door, and I'm like, "What about *my* needs, Miss?"

- DAVID CROSS

I believe the only time it's appropriate for a man to go with the strong belief that he should not stop and ask for directions is when he's looking for my G-Spot. No, you're not quite there yet. Maybe veer to the left? Oh, just keep going, you'll find it!

- NANCY PATTERSON

There are people so rich they don't get crabs, they get lobsters.

- ROBIN WILLIAMS

My mother sat us down one day and actually told us that masturbation could kill you. Ever since then I've been taking my life in own my hands.

- RAY ROMANO

In Germany a huge pile of porno magazines was discovered in the woods. They were found by a troop of boy scouts, three years ago.

- JAY LENO

A man on a date wonders if he'll get lucky. The woman knows.

- MONICA PIPER

With me, nothing works out. I bought a book *100 Ways to Make Love.* I ended up in traction. There was a misprint.

- RODNEY DANGERFIELD

Some men are heterosexual and some men are bisexual and some men don't think about sex at all... you know, they become lawyers.

- WOODY ALLEN

A study in a magazine asked men, "Would you rather the woman initiate sex?" Overwhelmingly, men said "Yes!" Women countered with the argument saying, "But every time we do, we get rejected and criticized." Welcome to the club.

- JACK COEN

How do you keep sex fresh? Put it in Tupperware.

- GARRY SHANDLING

Recently someone asked if I minded wearing a condom. *Au contraire*, I prefer them. There's no difference in the sensation, unless you count the total lack of any.

- RICHARD JENI

How come on the condom dispensers it has a little picture of birds flying over a pretty mountain? They use sex to sell everything else, why don't they use sex to sell condoms?

- JEFF CARNEGIE

The only thing my mother told me about sex was that I was never going to get any.

- DOUG GRAHAM

Researchers say Stonehenge was built in the form of the female sex organ. No wonder it's baffled men for five thousand years.

- JAY LENO

I met this transsexual at my gym and he was telling me about how he had a sex change to become a woman, and now he's started to date other women. I said, "Look, fellow/ma'am, I think you are making this a little bit harder than it has to be."

- SHASHI BHATIA

My husband and I tried really hard to have a baby, including having sex. But nothing happened. So we went to one of those fertility clinics where they charge you twelve million dollars every time your husband jerks off into a jar, but he was too uncomfortable there. Finally, to get a sample I had to fly him back home to his old room in his mother's house.

- KAREN HABER

The Kinsey Institute says gay men have bigger sex organs. Hence the origin of gay pride.

- JAY LENO

People who have intercourse with animals are offended by the term "bestiality"; they say it sounds brutal and uncaring. They prefer "Zoophile," lover of animals. Just let me repeat the amazing first part of that sentence: "People who have intercourse with animals are offended."

- DANIEL LIEBERT

I know my sexuality, but I get so confused by other people's. I don't even know the difference between transvestites and transsexuals. As I understand it, transvestites are the ones that grow down from the ceiling and transsexuals are the ones that grow up.

- PAMELA YAGER

How lucky we are that we can reach our genitals instead of that spot on our back that itches.

- FLASH ROSENBERG

A study claims that the relative lengths of the index and ring fingers indicates whether a woman is a lesbian. If between her thumb and index finger is another woman's nipple, that's an even better indication.

— BILL MAHER

People have always told me that I'd learn more from my kids than they'd learn from me. I believe that. I've learned that as a parent, when you have sex your body emits a hormone that drifts down the hall into your child's room and makes them want a drink of water.

— JEFF FOXWORTHY

A study shows college girls talk about sex at least as much as college guys. They just tell the truth.

— JAY LENO

It kills me the way they advertise phone sex: "Phone up and hear a woman's secret fantasies." If there's any reality to this, you'd hear stuff like, "Yeah, I'd like to be paid the same as a man for the same job."

- MIKE MACDONALD

This was in the news. A woman cut off her husband's penis while he was sleeping after she got a phone call from another woman. The worst part: the other woman had the wrong number.

- CONAN O'BRIEN

There are countries in the world where it's the custom for the men there to cut off a woman's clitoris. This is true and very gruesome. We should be happy that this will never happen in our country, because the men here don't know where the clitoris is.

- JANINE DITULLIO

The closest I ever came to a *ménage à trois* was once I dated a schizophrenic.

— RITA RUDNER

A survey asked married women when they most want to have sex. Eighty-four percent of them said right after their husband is finished.

— JAY LENO

I have tried a little kinky stuff. A woman called me and said, "I have mirrors all over my bedroom. Bring a bottle." I brought Windex.

— RODNEY DANGERFIELD

Heterosexuals are rude sometimes, get right in your face and ask you rude questions: "What do you lesbians do in bed?" Well, it's a lot like heterosexual sex. Only one of us doesn't have to fake an orgasm.

— SUZANNE WESTENHOEFER

Making love to a woman is like baking a turkey: You have to preheat the oven, stuff, baste, make some gravy, put it in for two hours, take it out; not done yet. Another hour, another hour. Finally it's ready. Men? It's microwave cooking. Rip off the package, three minutes: Ding! Gotta nap for an hour.

- CRAIG SHOEMAKER

A pitcher for the Cleveland Indians admits that he appeared in a gay porn film. Here's my question: When a guy's doing it with another guy are they both thinking of baseball?

- JAY LENO

I don't even understand how group sex works. What do they say afterwards? "Excuse me, was it good for anybody?"

- RITA RUDNER

I have one pick-up line which never works. If I'm at a club and I see a guy I like, I smile, and if he smiles back and I feel really comfortable I'll walk over and say, "Stick it in!"

- MARGARET CHO

When I got divorced, that was group sex. My wife screwed me in front of the jury.

- RODNEY DANGERFIELD

My mother said the best time to ask my dad for anything was during sex. Not the best advice I've ever been given.

- JIMMY CARR

Nobody's passing out condoms to increase the sexual activity of teenagers. Condoms don't make babies, people do.

- DENNIS MILLER

My husband wanted to spice up our love life with role play. He said, "I'll fulfill your fantasy, if you fulfill mine." I said, "Great, me first: Clean the bathtub."

- STEPHANIE BLUM

I want to show you my breasts and yet I'm frightened. I don't know what it is, but I touch them. They're fabulous. I had no idea. I think I'll go home with myself. Bye, gotta run. It's so great to be coy with your own body. "Hey, wanna go out?" "Get lost, scum. Beat it." Try spending the night alone with yourself sometime. You wake up the next morning, nobody will ever know what you were doing, not even you. "You wore me out. It was insane. I loved it."

- SANDRA BERNHARD

If I'm not in bed by eleven at night, I go home.

- HENNY YOUNGMAN

Mormons used to practice polygamy, but they outlawed it in 1890. So basically, they did away with the one thing that might entice most people to join their religion.

- STEVE NEAL

So I saw this ad in the paper, "Safe Sex Get Paid, Men 18-40." I call 'em up, it's a guidebook to sperm banks. And I'm thinking, why not get paid? I've done charity work for so long.

- NORMAN K.

A minor league pitcher for the Cleveland Indians apologized for appearing in a gay porn video. He said it was years ago, he was young, and he and his teammates needed money. So basically he took one for the team.

- JAY LENO

I understand that the doctor had to spank me when I was born, but I really don't see any reason he had to call me a whore.

– SARAH SILVERMAN

I have to compare the disadvantages of each: Marriage or not? Do I wanna go out every night talking about a bunch of stuff I'm not really interested in just to see if I can get some sex out of it? Or do I wanna be married, talking about a bunch of stuff I've heard before just to see if I can get some sex out of it?

– RICHARD JENI

You don't ever really want to visualize your parents having sex. It's very uncomfortable. Sex is a great thing and all. But you don't want to think that your whole life began because somebody had a little too much wine with dinner.

– JERRY SEINFELD

The women who got implants sued Dow Corning because they felt betrayed by their implant company. Betrayed? What, you mean I can't put a petroleum by-product in a baggie and insert it in my chest cavity safely? I am shocked! And betrayed!

- DANI KLEIN

I'm just a huge fan of the penis. Can I just say I love penises? They're just the greatest. And they're all different, like snowflakes.

- MARGARET CHO

Did you ever notice the people who are most adamantly against abortions are people so ugly you wouldn't want to touch them in the first place?

- GEORGE CARLIN

My old boyfriend used to say, "I read *Playboy* for the articles." Right, and I go to shopping malls for the music.

- RITA RUDNER

I tell ya how you can solve this abortion issue right now. Ready? Those unwanted babies that single moms leave in alleys and in dumpsters? Leave about twelve of those on the steps of the Supreme Court. It would be over, like that. "You guys said we had to have them? Then you guys can fucking raise them. You raise them. You said I had to have it? Then it's yours. It's yours, take it!"

- BILL HICKS

It was reported that sex is good for people with arthritis. It's just not that pleasant to watch.

- JAY LENO

A woman should dress to attract attention. To attract the most attention, a woman should be either nude or wearing something as expensive as getting her nude is going to be.

- P.J. O'ROURKE

I'd like to thank everyone who helped my parents conceive me: Grandma who babysat, Paul Masson for making Chablis cheap enough for my Pops to buy three bottles, Oldsmobile Cutlass Supreme for the roomy back seat which gave Pops the traction he needed to get into his love groove, and the pharmacist for supplying the defective prophylactic.

- ADAM SANDLER

A man in the Philippines whose wife accused him of infidelity cut off his own penis and handed it to her. It's a little slice of life story. Most guys won't even give up the remote.

- JAY LENO

Scientists say that chocolate affects your brain the same way sex does. Which means that after they eat a Snickers, guys roll over and go to sleep. And women ask the wrapper, "What are you thinking?"

- JIM WYATT

Who says we didn't have controversial subjects on TV back in my time? Remember Bonanza? It was about three guys in high heels living together.

- MILTON BERLE

Why do men name their penis? You hear them saying things like, "Well, Bobby's awake." You never hear women saying things like, "I'm sitting on Margaret."

- MARSHA WARFIELD

A study in Italy showed that people who eat a lot of pizza are less likely to get colon cancer. And another study says masturbation reduces risk of prostate cancer. It's what I've always said: diet and exercise.

— JAY LENO

I told my girlfriend that Dr. Ruth compared men to a sexual microwave: They start fast and finish fast. And women are more like crockpots: They take a long time to heat up, but can cook for hours. My girlfriend said, "Yeah, and you're like an old toaster that heats for ten seconds before it pops up."

— JOE DITZEL

There are a number of mechanical devices that increase sexual arousal, particularly in women. Chief amongst these is the Mercedes-Benz 380L convertible.

— P.J. O'ROURKE

Even though I'm single again, I'm still buying condoms. I don't want the woman at the store to think that I've stopped having sex. I don't really think that's any of her business. Although the condoms are piling up, so I'm going to have to have a lucky streak or think of a crafts project.

- JAKE JOHANNSEN

There ain't nothing an old man can do but bring me a message from a young one.

- MOMS MABLEY

Introductions are tricky in a lesbian relationship. It's a word game. To my friends she's my lover, to strangers and family members in denial she's my roommate, to Jehovah's Witnesses at the door she's my lesbian sex slave, and to my mother she's Jewish and that's all that matters.

- DENISE MCCANLES

A boob job is the gift that keeps on giving. My ex bought them, and my new guy enjoys them.

- ELAINE PELINO

A blood bank called the other day to see if I was interested in making a donation. For free. That just didn't seem right. Not when I'm still using my blood and I've got bills to pay. The sperm bank pays me for my generosity, even though we all know there's always plenty more where that came from. And the blood bank doesn't even let you keep their magazines. I know, because I asked.

- BRIAN BEATTY

In Germany, police are searching for a woman who holds men at gun point and forces them to have sex with her. Actually the gun isn't for the sex, it's to keep the guy around later to make him cuddle.

- JAY LENO

My ex-boyfriend had the nerve to call me up when he heard I was seeing someone else. He asked, "So, do you still think of me when you're having sex?" I said, "Honey, I didn't think of you when *we* were having sex."

- TRACY SMITH

My sister is a Disney freak. For Christmas she gave me their condoms. My favorite was the Mickey one, you know, because of the ears. And for the Pinocchio ones all I had to do was get my boyfriend to lie, which wasn't hard.

- PENNY WIGGINS

I actually learned about sex watching neighborhood dogs. And it was good. Go ahead and laugh. I think the most important thing I learned was: Never let go of the girl's leg no matter how hard she tries to shake you off.

- STEVE MARTIN

I talk to my wife while making love, if I happen to be near a phone.

- HENNY YOUNGMAN

According to *Psychology Today*, to keep your sex life active as a married couple, you should engage in role-playing. This works. Once a month my wife and I check into a cheap motel, and she pretends to be a hooker while I pretend to be a TV evangelist.

- WALLY WANG

Strippers are supposed to be a real macho thing to go see. I never understood this. Who was the first guy who wanted this? Somebody sitting around reading *Playboy*? "You know, this isn't frustrating enough, I'd like to see some live chicks I can't have."

- BOB NICKMAN

I have so much cyber sex, my baby's first words will be, "You've got mail."

- PAULARA R. HAWKINS

Premature ejaculation, I don't believe in that. If I cum, it was right on time, that's the way I see it. As far as I'm concerned I can't cum fast enough. They're mad at me because we have different goals in sex: I'm a speedfucker.

- DAVE CHAPELLE

Have you heard of this new book titled, *1,001 Sex Secrets Men Should Know*? It contains comments from 1,001 different women on how men can be better in bed. I think that women would actually settle for three: Slow down, turn off the TV, call out the right name.

- JAY LENO

More women believe in ghosts than men. They've had experience. They have sex with a guy. They turn around, and he's vanished.

- JAY LENO

If I ever wrote a sex manual, it would be called, *Ouch, You're on My Hair*.

- RICHARD LEWIS

Once the sexual revolution took hold, people really didn't have to buy the cow to get the milk. And girls today are like the dairy barn. So guys don't feel the necessity to get married. And the girls don't either.

- JOY BEHAR

Why do women go to tanning salons? What a waste of time and money. Guys only like the white parts, anyway.

- MARGOT BLACK

A man can produce sperm until he dies. But at least it's more fun than getting killed crossing the street.

> - STRANGE DE JIM

I don't think a woman should be a virgin before marriage. She should have had at least one other disappointing experience.

> - MAUREEN MURPHY

Playboy never wants you to think the pictures are posed. "We just happened to catch Kathy typing nude on top of a Volvo this morning."

> - ELAYNE BOOSLER

What is a date really, but a job interview that lasts all night? The only difference is that in not many job interviews is there a chance you'll wind up naked.

> - JERRY SEINFELD

I asked my girlfriend who she fantasized about while we were having sex, and she said, "I don't really have time."

- OWEN O'NEILL

In a new sex survey they found eight percent of people had sex four or more times a week. Now here's the interesting part. That number drops to two percent when you add the phrase, "With a partner."

- DAVID LETTERMAN

Last week the San Francisco Zoo had its annual Valentine's Day sex tour. They said bears would rather masturbate than have sex. That's why they get so mad when hikers surprise them. And when they break into campsites, they're not looking for food. They're looking for magazines.

- JAY LENO

There's a new roller coaster ride at Disney World, it's called the G-spot. There's never a line, because no one can find it.

- MEL FINE

Eagles mate while flying at eighty miles an hour. And when they start to drop, they don't stop until the act is completed. So it's not uncommon they both hit the ground and die. That's how committed they are. Boy, don't we feel like wimps for stopping to answer the phone? I don't know about you, but if I'm one of those birds and we're getting close to the ground, I would seriously consider faking it.

- ELLEN DEGENERES

Two guys in a health club, one is putting on pantyhose. "Since when do you wear pantyhose?" one asks. "Since my wife found them in the glove compartment of my car."

- HENNY YOUNGMAN

The Discovery Channel had a fascinating show on the mating habits of hyenas. They said that the male hyena often will get angry at the female hyena while they are having sex. It doesn't help that the female hyena is laughing at you all the time.

- JAY LENO

I was once involved in a same-sex marriage. There was the same sex over and over and over.

- DAVID LETTERMAN

Everyone loves Hershey's Kisses and Hugs. I'm waiting for Hershey's Gropes.

- MYQ KAPLAN

Movie Indians say, "White man speak with forked tongue." I wish! If I had a forked tongue I'd use it, I'd be scraping satisfied women off my bedroom ceiling with a spatula.

- DANIEL LIEBERT

I took my wife out for her birthday. I made a toast: "To the best woman a man ever had." The waiter joined in.

- RODNEY DANGERFIELD

There are all these magazine articles pushing the joys of senior sex. Oh sure, especially for my mother. "Can you try not to move much? I have vertigo and tend to get dizzy very easily. And we should leave some water by the bed because my medication makes me dehydrated. Can my aide stay in the room in case I need to get up during the act?"

- JUDY GOLD

Men only have two feelings, we're either hungry or horny. I tell my wife, if I don't have an erection, make me a sandwich.

- BOBBY SLAYTON

My girlfriend buys generic products that worry me. For instance, the generic "I Can't Believe it's Not I Can't Believe it's Not Butter" bothers me because it's butter twice removed. And then there's her generic birth control, "Hey, What Are the Odds?"

– DERIC HARRINGTON

It's spicier having sex with your ex-wife isn't it? It's like you're cheating on yourself.

– TOM ARNOLD

For the holidays here in Los Angeles, women are getting snow globe breast implants. When they jiggle it looks like it's snowing.

– JAY LENO

I want Baskin-Robbins to develop a cone that licks back.

– JOHNNY CARSON

If I have phone sex to avoid getting pregnant, is that caller IUD?

- MARGOT BLACK

The other night I went into a gay bar. It was ridiculous. There were fifteen guys for every guy.

- RODNEY DANGERFIELD

The guys in strip clubs think because they got a pocket full of dollars they got the power, but the chicks got the power. They spin around the pole and you guys are hypnotized. That's how I look at a dessert case, but at least I get to eat mine.

- MONIQUE MARVEZ

An aphrodisiac is a drug two people take, and then both pretend it worked.

- STRANGE DE JIM

I spent five years in the Air Force, and if it wasn't for sexual harassment no one would have talked to me at all. An officer accused me of being a lesbian. I would have denied it, but I was lying naked on top of her at the time.

- LYNDA MONTGOMERY

Can you imagine what a nightmare it must have been before they invented painkillers? What did they do, have a guy bite a bullet? They could have done better than that. Bring in a big-breasted woman. That would distract any man. Stick a knife through their arm, they see those big breasts, they don't feel a thing.

- JOY BEHAR

I know nothing about relationships because I went to Catholic school, where Sex Ed classes were taught by nuns. That's like taking your car to an Amish mechanic.

- JEFFREY JENA

It was one of those bachelor parties where all the married men had to meet at the end and decide about what to say we did, "We got in a fight with some guys and that's how our underwear got ripped. They ripped our underwear, and smelled good. Jimmy, you fell and your nipple got pierced."

— RAY ROMANO

I wanted to show my cooking group an instructional show on TV, so I ordered the Spice Channel. It started out okay. There was a woman baking a cake and then a man came into the picture, and let me just say for the record that I have never seen a cake frosted that way.

— MARY GALLAGHER

According to a new survey, fifty-six percent of women carry condoms. The other forty-four percent are carrying babies.

— JAY LENO

I saw the movie "Jackass" and the feminist in me was offended there weren't any women participating in the stupid stunts. But then I realized there are already women doing jackass stuff on videotape. It's called porn.

- WENDY WILKINS

The Supreme Court has ruled that sex between two men is legal, and sex between two women is exciting.

- CONAN O'BRIEN

I overheard these two young guys talking about women and sex. One guy says, "It's so much easier for women to have an orgasm on top." And the other guy argued, "No, it's easier for women to have an orgasm when she's on the bottom." Finally, I turned to them and said, "Guys, actually it's much easier when we're alone."

- CORY KAHANEY

I have French doors in the bedroom. They don't open unless I lick them.

- *JUDY GOLD*

A study shows that the more female friends a man has, the less likely he is to have a heart attack, unless his wife catches him with them.

- *JAY LENO*

I'm not into that one-night thing. I think a person should get to know someone, and even be in love with them, before you use them and degrade them.

- *STEVE MARTIN*

If they can put a man on the moon, why can't they put one in me?

- *FLASH ROSENBERG*

People in different parts of the world react differently after sex. A German woman is practical. She will say, *"Ach, dat vas goot!"* A French woman is solicitous. She will say, *"Ah, mon cherie*, did I please you?" and an English woman will say, "Feeling better?"

- GODFREY CAMBRIDGE

My wife wants Olympic sex, once every four years.

- RODNEY DANGERFIELD

I meet guys who absolutely have no concept of monogamy, they think it's a game by Milton Bradley.

- CATHY LADMAN

Zoos are starting to give contraceptives to their animals. I can barely open a condom, and *I* have thumbs.

- CRAIG KILBORN

A girl's legs are her best friends, but the best of friends must part.

- REDD FOXX

Don't cook. Don't clean. No man will ever make love to a woman because she waxed the linoleum. "My God, the floor's immaculate. Lie down, you hot bitch."

- JOAN RIVERS

Today I was reading about the North American Nude Bikers Association. It's bad enough when a flying bug hits you in the face.

- JAY LENO

Sex when you're married is like going to the 7-Eleven: There's not much variety, but at three in the morning, it's always there.

- CAROL LEIFER

Some people say older men have long endurance and can make love longer. Let's think about this: Who wants to fuck an old man for a long time?

- MARSHA WARFIELD

It wasn't easy telling my family that I'm gay. I made my carefully worded announcement at Thanksgiving. I said, "Mom, would you please pass the gravy to a homosexual?" She passed it to my father.

- BOB SMITH

San Francisco is going to pay for city employees who want sex changes. The city will save money, though. After they change a man to a woman, they only have to pay her seventy-five percent of what he was making. The HMO version is a sock to stuff down your pants, and a remote control. "OK, you're a guy."

- JAY LENO

Men think sex is their idea. How stupid of us. Women have already decided when, where, who, and how many times. Guys think if we get a woman drunk she'll say yes. Bull! She's already decided yes, getting drunk is a bonus.

- BOB DUBAC

My uncle got a vasectomy. Put it on MasterCard. Forgot to pay. The finance company came over and knocked up his wife.

- ELAYNE BOOSLER

The only perfect man is Mr. Ed. He's hung like a horse, and can hold a conversation.

- TRACI SKENE

You know what I like more than women? Pornography. Because I can get pornography.

- PATTON OSWALT

Sex is simple, once you realize it's just like riding a bicycle. In both cases, the hardest part is learning not to fall off.

- STRANGE DE JIM

I wanted to make it really special on Valentine's Day, so I tied my boyfriend up. And for three solid hours I watched whatever I wanted to on TV.

- TRACY SMITH

In Ohio, a sixth-grade boy was suspended for three days for bringing the *Sports Illustrated* swimsuit issue to school with him. That's how you punish a 13-year-old boy: Send him home for three days with the *Sports Illustrated* swimsuit issue? Then what, lock him in the bathroom?

- JAY LENO

I'm not an advocate of three-way sex. They're like that Lucy episode where Lucy and Ethel are trying to stuff all the chocolate into their mouths. I tried a five-way once, but I'm too needy. Afterwards I was like, "So are we all in a relationship now?"

– MARGARET CHO

Before we got married, my wife told me I was one in a million. I found out she was right.

– RODNEY DANGERFIELD

My wife left me, I should have seen it coming. For the past year she called me her "insignificant other." By the end of the marriage her favorite position was man on top, woman visiting her mother. When we did actually do it, we only did it doggie-style so we could both watch the weather channel.

– DANIEL LIEBERT

Have you ever been drunk and making out with someone and you just feel like kissing, and he pulls his package out? I didn't ask for that. The way that I dealt with it was I just put my hand on it and left it there, very awkward. But I was remembering one time when I was a kid and my parents asked my brother to do the dishes, and he just did them very badly, so they never asked him to do it again.

- MARTHA KELLY

You know what's the worst contraceptive? The Pill. Because you have to keep taking it every day, regardless of what's going on in your love life. It's so nice during those two-year lulls to have a daily reminder. "I sleep alone, but oh my, look, it's time for my loser pill." Can you imagine if men had to wear a condom for 30 days just in case they might need it? "It's day 28, but somebody might call."

- CAROLINE RHEA

When you want your husband to play with you, wear a full-length black nightgown with buttons all over it. Sure, it's uncomfortable, but it makes you look just like his remote control.

- DIANA JORDAN

I have heard women say they can judge how a guy will be in bed from how he dances. I hope that's not true. Because I come from rednecks, and my people invented square dancing. Which means we're so bad at it, we have to have someone tell us what to do, as we're doing it.

- STEVE NEAL

According to a study in *McCall's* magazine, the sexiest thing a man can say to a woman is, "Let me do the dishes." This is what I hate about these magazines, they set impossible standards.

- JAY LENO

I don't understand the *Sports Illustrated* swimsuit issue. Bikini models in a magazine about sports? That'll make sense the day I see Dick Butkus in the Victoria's Secret catalogue.

- SHEILA WENZ

I don't think anyone should get up early in the morning. Nothing good ever happens in the morning. Have you ever observed people in the morning? They tend to be flossing, scratching or eating things like boiled eggs. At night, you drink fine wine and make love, neither of which requires flossing.

- RICHARD JENI

My psychologist told me that a lot of men suffer from premature ejaculation. That's not true, women suffer.

- ROBERT SCHIMMEL

According to a new survey, seventy-six percent of men would rather watch a football game than have sex. My question is, why do we have to choose? Why do you think they invented half-time?

— *JAY LENO*

I have low self-esteem. When we were in bed together, I would fantasize that I was someone else.

— *RICHARD LEWIS*

Beverly Hills requires that stores put this label on all fur coats: "Warning: Your husband is having an affair."

— *CRAIG KILBORN*

I don't get no respect. I went to a massage parlor. It was self service.

— *RODNEY DANGERFIELD*

I love blowjobs because they involve my two favorite things: cumming, and doing nothing.

- ADAM RICHMOND

I asked my wife, "On a scale of one to ten, how do you rate me as a lover?" She said, "You know I'm no good at fractions."

- RODNEY DANGERFIELD

A professor at the University of Kansas is in trouble for showing x-rated videos in his class. And his class was algebra.

- JAY LENO

Men are like flowers. If you don't know how to handle a rose, you get stuck by a couple of pricks.

- MARGOT BLACK

When my wife has sex with me there's always a reason. One night she used me to time an egg.

- RODNEY DANGERFIELD

We noticed that the bride was pregnant. So at the wedding everyone threw puffed rice.

- DICK CAVETT

When my teenage daughter told us that her Sex Education teacher had demonstrated how to put on a condom, my wife asked, "On what? A cucumber? Boy, are they letting you in for a big disappointment."

- ROBERT SCHIMMEL

A woman escaped death when a bullet shot by her jealous husband lodged in her breast implant. And I almost lost a thumb.

- CRAIG KILBORN

I know women can fantasize, but, oh, they have no idea what men are capable of. We have a cast of thousands in our head.

- RAY ROMANO

The stick insect has sex for 79 days straight. If it's only been 77 days, is that a quickie? And you know that even after 79 days, the female goes, "Oh, so close!" And the guy tells his buddies it was 158 days.

- JAY LENO

The newlyweds were married five days. He turns to her and says, "Honey, we're gonna make love a new way tonight. We're gonna lie back to back." She says, "How can that be any fun?" He says, "I've invited another couple."

- WOODY WOODBURY

I went to the Erotic Bakery today and got something that really turned my lady on: A cake in the shape of my wallet.

- CRAIG KILBORN

Women are really not that exacting. They only desire one thing in bed. Take off your socks. And by the way, they're not going to invite their best girlfriend over for a three-some, so you can stop asking.

- DENNIS MILLER

Men are delusional. Hugh Hefner lounges around in a bathrobe with three live-in girlfriends. You know guys are sitting at home watching the Playboy Channel and thinking, "That could be me. I've got a bathrobe."

- DENISE MUNRO ROBB

Republicans are upset that federal funds are being used by the Kinsey Institute to study sexual arousal. Republicans are against using federal funds to study sexual arousal unless the study leads to impeachment.

- JAY LENO

There exists a widespread folk myth that humans should learn about sex from their parents. My relationship with my father nearly ended when he tried to teach me how to drive. I can't imagine our relationship having survived his instructing me how to operate my penis.

- BOB SMITH

I'm a bad lover. Once I caught a Peeping Tom booing me.

- RODNEY DANGERFIELD

I'm getting more and more inconsiderate. I slept with a young guy and afterward I said, "That was fun. It's been so long since I've slept with someone for a ride home."

– LAURA KIGHTLINGER

I'm so sick of men saying that women have all the power, because men are slaves to their penis. What you mean is that the one percent of women who look like *Playboy* centerfolds can get you to do anything, and the other 99% of us can't get a tire changed at rush hour. "Excuse me, sir? Oh, I guess he's gotta go home to log on at the Pamela Anderson web site."

– ANN OELSCHLAGER

When a masochist brings someone home from a bar, does he say, "Excuse me a moment, I'm going to slip into something uncomfortable"?

– GEORGE CARLIN

That seventh-grade teacher had sex with one of her students twenty times. Well, that's how kids learn, repetition.

- JAY LENO

My mother said not to go to bars to meet people. Go to a place like a museum. So I went there and I stood in the middle of a room full of paintings and I screamed, "Somebody fuck me!"

- ROBIN RYAN

Our honeymoon night was hot. My wife was moaning all night in ecstasy, opening gifts. "An orange squeezer! Oh my God! A waffle maker!" Next morning the guy down the hall gave me the big thumbs-up. "Boy, you were using everything but the kitchen sink in there."

- MIKE BINDER

For guys sex is like going to a restaurant. No matter what they order off that menu, they walk out saying, "Damn, that was good!" For women it don't work like that. We go to the restaurant, sometimes it's good, sometimes we got to send it back. You have those hit and misses, you might want to skip a few meals. Or you might go, "I think I'm going to cook for myself today."

- WANDA SYKES

I dropped all my Viagra pills in the toilet. Now the lid won't go down.

- RODNEY DANGERFIELD

Apparently in some states you're now going to be able to vote on the Internet. I don't think I want people voting on the Internet, knowing what they do. Because you'll get candidates saying things like, "Ask yourself this, are you getting off now better than you were four years ago?"

- BILL MAHER

In an article in *Newsweek* I noticed the phrase "sexually illiterate." I didn't understand. Does anybody's penis read? Mine doesn't. It will look at pictures. But I have never seen it yawn and put a bookmark in.

- GARRY SHANDLING

A study showed attractive men produce the best quality sperm. I'd think it would be unattractive men. They produce it by hand.

- JAY LENO

I really hate it when strange men on the street say, "Smile! You'd look so much prettier if you'd smile." I always feel like saying, "Get hard! You'd look so much more useful if you had an erection."

- CATHYRN MICHON

My Uncle Norman is a Mormon. He lives in Utah. He was married to three women at once. The third one turned out to be a militant lesbian. She sued him for divorce and got custody of the other two.

- DINO LONDIS

The basic conflict between men and women sexually is that men are like firemen. To us, sex is an emergency, and no matter what we're doing we can be ready in two minutes. Women are like fire. They're very exciting, but the conditions have to be exactly right for it to occur.

- JERRY SEINFELD

It's silly for a woman to go to a male gynecologist. It's like going to an auto mechanic who has never owned a car.

- CARRIE SNOW

GREEN ROOM

Woody Allen is a comedian, actor and Academy Award-winning director of several films, including *Annie Hall* and *Mighty Aphrodite*.

Tom Arnold is a comedian and actor who appeared in the movies *True Lies* and *Nine Months*. Arnold is currently a co-host on Fox Sports Net's *The Best Damn Sports Show Period*.
   Web site: tomarnoldonline.com

Dave Attell has been a writer for *Saturday Night Live*, nominated for an American Comedy Award, and is currently the star of Comedy Central's *Insomniac*.

Comedian **Michele Balan** has appeared on Comedy Central, USA Network and Lifetime TV.
   Web site: michelebalan.com

Roseanne Barr is the comedian who has specialized in the eponymous TV shows *Roseanne* the sitcom, *The Roseanne Show* talk show, and *The Real Roseanne Show* reality show.
   Web site: roseanneworld.com

Dave Barry is the author of a bazillion humor books, including *The World According To Dave Barry*.
   Web site: davebarry.com

Joy Behar is a comedian and actress who serves as comic relief on the ABC daytime talk show *The View*.

Brian Beatty is a writer and comedian in Minneapolis whose articles and reviews have appeared in *Blues Revue, Guitar World Acoustic, Minnesota Monthly, Publishers Weekly, The Rake* and *Seventeen*. His jokes have also appeared on the BBC comedy Web site. He's taller than he is wide.
   Contact: brianbeatty@lycos.com

Doug Benson is a stand-up comedian and actor who has appeared on *Jimmy Kimmel Live, Comedy Central Presents, Friends* and *Yes, Dear*. Benson is also agent provocateur of the hit off-Broadway show *The Marijuana-Logues*.

Milton Berle was a comedian who popularized TV with his early 1950s comedy show and went on to numberless appearances on the *Ed Sullivan Show* and the *Tonight Show*. Berle also starred in movies that include *It's a Mad, Mad, Mad, Mad World*.

Comedian **Sandra Bernhard** co-starred on the sitcom *Roseanne* and has appeared in a number of films, which include *The King of Comedy*.
  Web site: sandrabernhard.com

Comedian **Shashi Bhatia** has appeared as a host on the Sci Fi Channel, on the sitcoms *Friends* and *Seinfeld*, and in the movie *Leaving Las Vegas*.
  Contact: ShashiBhatia@hotmail.com

Mike Binder is a comedian, screenwriter, and director of the critically acclaimed film, *The Upside of Anger*.
  Web site: mikebinder.net

In 1975, **Rob Bitter** was voted "Most-Talented Seventh-Grader" at Beck Middle School in Cherry Hill, New Jersey.
  Contact: thenumberthirteen@yahoo.com

Comedian **Lewis Black** is a political correspondent and curmudgeon for *The Daily Show*.
  Web site: lewisblack.net

Comedian **Margot Black** is a writer, producer and stand-up comedian whose credits include MTV's *Jenny McCarthy Show* and *Late Night with David Letterman*.
  Web site: margotblack.com

Comedian **Ed Bluestone** is a 1970s comedian who segued to book author. He was also known for having created the best-selling *National Lampoon* cover "Buy This Magazine or We'll Shoot This Dog."

Comedian **Stephanie Blum** took first prize in the Ladies of Laughter Funniest Female competition at Madison Square Garden, was chosen by HBO's US Comedy Arts Festival to be their 2003 "Breakout Performer," and also is a *Star Search* winner.
    Web site: actoneentertainment.net/comedian_44.html

Comedian **Elayne Boosler** has starred in her own HBO and Showtime specials, including *Party of One*. She is currently the host of PAX TV's *Balderdash*.
    Web site: elayneboosler.com

Alicia Brandt is a stand-up comedian and an actress who has appeared in a range of roles from the soap opera *General Hospital* to the movie *Mousehunt*.

Comedian **Bill Braudis** has appeared on *Late Night with Conan O'Brien*.

Judy Brown is the editor of this book.
    Web site: judybrown.info
    Contact: judybrowni@usa.net

George Burns was a classic comedian whose career stretched from vaudeville to the 1950s sitcom *Burns and Allen*, and the 1970s movie *Oh, God*.

Comedian **Brett Butler** has been the star of the sitcom *Grace Under Fire*.
    Web site: brettbutler.com

Red Buttons was a composer, comedian, author and actor whose films include *Sayonara*.

Godfrey Cambridge was an African American actor and comedian whose style was drawn off the racial climate of the 1950s and 1960s. One of his most memorable roles was in the 1970 film *Watermelon Man*, in which he played a white man who turned black overnight.

Drew Carey is, coincidentally enough, the star of the now-syndicated *The Drew Carey Show*. Carey is also executive producer and host of the comedy improv show *Who's Line is it Anyway?*

Comedian **George Carlin** has won a Grammy, a CableAce award and was nominated for an Emmy for his comedy albums, HBO, and network comedy specials.
Web site: georgecarlin.com

Jeff Carnegie is a humor writer.

British comedian **Jimmy Carr** is a Perrier Award nominee, the Time Out Award winner for Best Stand-up and the Royal Television Society award winner for Best On-Screen Newcomer.
Web site: jimmycarr.com

Johnny Carson, the "King of Late Night TV," hosted NBC's *Tonight Show* for more than thirty years.

Comedian **Judy Carter** is the author of the book *The Comedy Bible* but bills herself as "just another Jewish lesbian comic-magician."
Web site: judycarter.com

Dick Cavett parlayed a 1960s stand-up comedy career into a series of his own talk shows on network, PBS and cable.

It stands to reason that Comedian **Dave Chappelle** is the host of *Chappelle's Show* on Comedy Central.
Web site: davechappelle.com

Comedian **Margaret Cho**, the comedy diva, is the star of her own stand-up films including *I'm the One That I Want*, *Notorious C.H.O.* and *Revolution*.
Web site: margaretcho.com

Kate Clinton is a ground-breaking lesbian stand-up comedian whose career spans three decades. Her comedy albums include *Babes in Joyland, Read My Lips*, and *The Marrying Kind*.
Web site: kateclinton.com

Comedian **Jack Coen** has made a dozen appearances on the *Tonight Show* and, no fools they, they made him a staff writer. He also recently starred in his own Comedy Central special.

Bobby Collins has starred in his own Showtime special, been host of VH1's *Stand-up Spotlight*, and produced the comedy CDs *On The Inside*, and the Grammy-nominated *Out Of Bounds*.
Web site: bobbycollins.com

Scotland's favorite comedian, **Billy Connolly**, has been featured in several films, including his star turn in both *Her Majesty, Mrs. Brown* and *Man Who Sued God*.
Web site: billyconnolly.com

Comedian **David Corrado**, who performs throughout Los Angeles, also writes for several comedians.
Contact: dcorrado@ucla.edu

Comedian **Wayne Cotter** hosted the Fox television series *Comic Strip Live* every Saturday night for three years. He also appears regularly on the *Late Show with David Letterman* and the *Tonight Show with Jay Leno*.
Web site: waynecotter.com

The Covert Comic is an actual CIA officer who likes to write intelligence jokes and prose, post them on his Web site, and donate the proceeds to U.S. veterans and their families.
Web site: covertcomic.com

Comedian **David Cross** is half of the team who instigated HBO's *Mr. Show,* but is wholly responsible for his CDs *Shut Up You Fucking Baby!* and *It's Not Funny.*
   Web site: bobanddavid.com

Comedian **Billy Crystal** is an actor, writer, producer and director. His movies include *City Slickers* and *When Harry Met Sally.* Crystal has also hosted the Academy Awards.

Comedian **Michael Dane** has been entertaining audiences for fifteen years, everywhere from Seattle to Maine, as a stand-up comedian and with his solo show *No Apparent Motive.* He also created the Gay and Lesbian Comedy Night at the Comedy Store in Hollywood.

Comedian **Rodney Dangerfield** was the star of several movies including *Caddyshack, Back to School* and improbably enough, *Natural Born Killers.* He also won a Grammy for his comedy album *No Respect.*
   Web site: rodney.com

Beth Davidoff is a stand-up comedian, writer, and stay-at-home mom who lives in Las Vegas.
   Web site: comedy.com/bethd

Comedian **Ellen DeGeneres** is the groundbreaking star of the ABC sitcom *Ellen,* and has been featured in movies that include *Love Letters* and *Mr. Wrong.* She has made a home for herself in the daytime arena with her hit syndicated talk show, *The Ellen DeGeneres Show,* which won four Emmys in its first year alone.

Tony Deyo is a stand-up comic from High Point, North Carolina.
   Web site: tonydeyo.com

Kathie Dice, a comedian, wife, mother, and hairdresser, to boot, has also written and performed her own one-woman show, *I'm Just Me...Mary,* a humorous look at the life of the Virgin Mary.
   Web site: kjthedj.homestead.com/mary.html

Phyllis Diller is one of the first women stand-up comedians to go professional in the 1950s. Her nearly fifty-year career included a number of movies and dozens of TV shows, including appearances on the *Tonight Show*.

Comedian **Janine DiTullio** has been a staff writer for *Late Night with Conan O'Brien* and *The Daily Show with Jon Stewart*.

Comedian **Joe Ditzel** is the editor of the book, *Best of the Net Wits*, and his own weekly humor column, which is syndicated at his Web site.
    Web site: joeditzel.com

Comedian **Tom Dreesen** has performed extensively in a three-decade comedy career including in Las Vegas, on the *Tonight Show*, and as an opening act for Elvis Presley and Frank Sinatra.
    Web site: tomdreesen.com

Comedian **Bob Dubac** has bridged a career between acting, comedy and writing for over ten years. In a desire to bring the three together, Dubac created and starred in his one-man show, *The Male Intellect: an Oxymoron*?
    Web site: maleintellect.com

Political comedian and five-time Emmy nominee **Will Durst** is host/co-producer of the award-winning PBS series *Livelyhood*. Durst has also appeared on the *Late Show with David Letterman*, Comedy Central, HBO, and Showtime.
    Web site: willdurst.com

Comedian **Bil Dwyer** is the host of *Extreme Dodgeball* and *Battlebots*. He has also appeared on *Ally McBeal*, *The Larry Sanders Show*, Comedy Central, and the *Late Late Show with Craig Kilborn*.

Chris Elliot has starred in the movie *Cabin Boy* and the sitcom *Get a Life*, and also plays a recurring character on *Everybody Loves Raymond*.

Leah Eva is a San Francisco-based stand-up comedian who tells us she also hopes be the first Filipina-American to have more shoes than Imelda Marcos.
    Contact: leahsmillions@aol.com

Comedian **Jennifer Fairbanks** has performed on UPN's *Vibe*, and is also a member of the comedy troupe Fresh Meat, an award-winning San Francisco improv group.

Jimmy Fallon has been a featured player on *Saturday Night Live* and co-anchor of "Weekend Update." He has recently turned to the big screen, starring in the action/comedy *Taxi*.
    Web site: jimmyfallon.net

A father of five, **Ken Ferguson** performs comedy in the Midwest. "I need to tell the world how ticked off I am, and make people laugh at the same time."
    Web site: kenferguson.net

Tina Fey is co-anchor of *Saturday Night Live*'s "Weekend Update." Fey debuted as a screenwriter with the wildly popular movie *Mean Girls*.

Mel Fine is a working comedian throughout the Midwest, and the winner of the Indianapolis Funniest Person Contest.

Redd Foxx was a stand-up comedian for over forty years and the star of the 1970s sitcom *Sanford and Son*.

Jeff Foxworthy is known both for his former eponymous sitcom and *You Might Be a Redneck If*, "the biggest-selling comedy album of all time." Foxworthy recently released a new CD, *Big Funny*, and hosts Comedy Central's *Blue Collar Comedy*.
    Web site: jefffoxworthy.com

Comedian **Catherine Franco** has played leading ladies in heavy theatrical shows such as *Extremities* and *Children of a Lesser God*, home-wrecking bitches in a dozen soap operas, and now performs in comedy clubs that include the Laugh Factory in Los Angeles.
    Web site: catherinefranco.com

Mary Gallagher is an actress and comedian whose television credits include *Friends* and the *Tonight Show*.
    Web site: marygallagher.tv

Comedian **Zach Galifiniakis** has written for *That '70s Show* and briefly hosted the *Late World with Zach* talk show.

Comedian **Emmy Gay** has appeared at both the Apollo Theater and the Joseph Papp Public Theater. She has created and toured several one-person shows including *Nappy Hair a Celebration of Diversity*.
    Web site: emmygay.com

Comedian **Tina Georgie** has appeared on the *Late Late Show with Craig Kilborn*.

Irv Gilman is a comedian, MC and former Council Member of Monterey Park, California.

Comedian **Judy Gold** is the host of HBO's *At the Multiplex with Judy Gold* and a regular fixture on Comedy Central, *The View*, and VH1. Judy has also won two Emmy Awards for writing and producing *The Rosie O'Donnell Show*.
    Web site: judygold.com

Bob Goldthwait has starred in movies, including *Scrooged*, and on TV series that include *Unhappily Ever After*. Bob has also directed the movie *Shakes the Clown*, and *Chapelle's Show* on Comedy Central.

Mimi Gonzalez produced the weekly stand-up show *Women with Balls* for six years in Los Angeles and San Francisco. Mimi has also performed comedy from Wenatchee to Biloxi, Tallahasee to Albany, and counts entertaining the troops in Japan, Korea, Bosnia and Kosovo as some of her most rewarding work.
Web site: mimigonzalez.com

A touring headliner, **Reno Goodale** has been seen on the TV shows *Sunday Comics, Stand-Up Stand-Up, Short Attention Span Theatre,* and in numerous commercials. Goodale has also written jokes for comedians, including Jay Leno, and has been quoted in the *Los Angeles Times'* "Laugh Lines."

Comedian **Doug Graham** has opened for many national acts including Drew Carey, Kevin Meaney, Phoebe Snow, and Spyrogyra.
Web site: comedygraham.com

Comedian **Kathy Griffin** has been featured in the sitcom *Suddenly Susan* as well as the reality programs *Celebrity Mole* and *Average Joe.* She currently stars in her stand-up comedy special, *The D List,* which can be seen on Bravo.
Web site: kathygriffin.net

Matt Groening is the executive producer, writer and creator of *The Simpsons* and *Futurama.*
Web site: mattgroening.com

Mark Gross is a comedy writer and comedian who has written for *Politically Incorrect with Bill Maher* and appeared on the *Tonight Show with Jay Leno, Late Friday,* and Comedy Central's *Premium Blend.*
Web site: markgrosscomedy.com

Comedian **Karen Haber** has been featured on the *Arsenio Hall Show, Evening at the Improv,* and in the video *The Girls of the Comedy Store.*

Deric Harrington is a comedian who likes his Web site and the taste of victory.
   Web site: dericharrington.com

Paulara R. Hawkins has been a semi-finalist in Comedy Central's Laugh Riot Competition, and been featured as one of the Comedians to Watch on *The Jenny Jones Show*.
   Web site: artistwebsite.com/paularapage.html

Cindy Heidel has performed at the Natural Fudge in Hollywood.

Janice Heiss is a comedian and member of the San Francisco theater group The Plutonium Players. Her writing has appeared in the literary magazine, *Passages North* and the books *Herotica 2* and *The Ecstatic Moment: the Best of Libido*.

Comedian **Carol Henry** has been featured in HBO's *Women of the Night III*.

In the 1980s and early 1990s **Bill Hicks** made eleven appearances on *Late Night with David Letterman*, and released his first concert video, *Sane Man*. Hicks recorded four comedy albums during his lifetime (including *Dangerous* and *Relentless*). Two more albums, *Arizona Bay* and *Rant in E-Minor*, were issued posthumously.

Bob Hope was a comedian whose career ranged over seven decades, from vaudeville, to a series of "Road" movies with Bing Crosby, and innumerable television specials.

Eric Idle, most famously of the Monty Python troupe and the movie *Life of Brian*, is also creator of the Python Broadway musical *Spamalot*.

Tony Invergo is a comedian and magician who's been performing since 1988 in the United States and Europe. He currently makes his home and works in Illinois.
   Contact: uncent@hotmail.com

Jeffrey Jena is a writer and stand-up comic who has appeared on over thirty national television shows. Jeff is a regular guest on the *Bob and Tom* Radio program.
Web site: jeffreyjena.com

Comedian **Richard Jeni** has been rewarded for his comic fluidity with two CableAce Awards and one American Comedy Award. He has also made his mark as the star of his own TV show, an actor in feature films, and an award-winning TV host.
Web site: richardjeni.com

Comedian **Jake Johannsen** has starred in two HBO specials, made over 30 appearances on *Late Night with David Letterman* and released the CD *Live at Cobb's Comedy Club*.
Web site: jakethis.com

Comedian **Jenny Jones** just completed a successful 12-year run as host of the nationally syndicated talk show *The Jenny Jones Show*. Jones previously became the first woman to win the *Star Search* comedy grand prize, and afterwards, developed a revolutionary comedy show *Girls Night Out*.
Web site: jennyjones.com

Comedian **Diana Jordan** has been nominated for an American Comedy Award, has appeared in the movie *Jerry McGuire*, and authored the bestselling book *A Wife's Little Instruction Book: Your Survival Guide to Marriage without Bloodshed*.
Web site: dianajordan.com

Comedian **Norman K.** performs at clubs in the New York area.
Contact: normank_comic@hotmail.com

Comedian **Cory Kahaney** was a finalist in the first season of NBC's *Last Comic Standing*. She has appeared on *Comedy Central Presents, Tough Crowd with Colin Quinn, Politically Incorrect with Bill Mahar*, Lifetime's *Girls Night Out*, and NBC's *Comedy Showcase*.
Web site: corykahaney.com

Comedian **Bill Kalmenson** has appeared in the movie *Lethal Weapon* and is the screenwriter and director of the film *The Souler Opposite*.

Jackie Kannon is a 1950s comedian whose record albums include *Live from the Ratfink Room* and *Songs for the John*.

Myq Kaplan performs music and comedy in the Boston area, is a regular at the Comedy Studio, and an irregular elsewhere. His CD is titled *Open Myq Night*.
    Web site: myqkaplan.com

Jonathan Katz created and stared in Comedy Central's *Dr. Katz, Professional Therapist*. He is also the author of the book *To Do Lists of the Dead*.

American Comedy Award nominee **Sheila Kay** is a regular on the comedy shows *Evening at the Improv, Make Me Laugh*, and *Stand-Up Spotlight*. Kay is currently touring in *Venus Attacks*, a comedy about love, sex, and self-help.
    Web site: sheilakay.com

Comedian **Martha Kelly** has appeared on Comedy Central, and featured on NBC's *Last Comic Standing*.

Comedian **Jen Kerwin** has appeared on NBC's *Last Comic Standing*.

In addition to being comedy's reigning Queen of Sardonica, comedian **Laura Kightlinger** is also a writer and producer of the sitcom *Will and Grace*.

Comedian **Craig Kilborn** has been the host of CBS's *The Late Late Show*, and made appearances in feature films, including *Old School*.

Dani Klein is a comedian and actor who has appeared on *Law and Order*, and the remake of the film *The Out of Towners*.

Besides appearing the *Tonight Show* a bazillion times, comedian **Cathy Ladman** was a writer and recurring character on *Caroline in the City*. She has also made appearances on *Just Shoot Me* and *Everybody Loves Raymond*.

Since moving back to San Antonio, **Todd Larson**'s unique style of sarcastic, relatable humor has made him an audience favorite throughout Texas. Performing regularly at the Rivercenter Comedy Club, Todd has worked with many talented comedians such as Chris Fonseca and Shawn Gnandt.
  Contact: acelarson@aol.com

Lynn Lavner has taken her original brand of music and comedy to forty-one states and seven countries. Her albums include *Butch Fatale* and *You are What You Wear*.

Okay, she's not a comedian, but **Fran Lebowitz** is the incisively witty author of the books *Metropolitan Life* and *The Fran Lebowitz Reader*.

Comedian **James Leemer** has appeared on Comedy Central.

Comedian **Carol Leifer** has been a producer on *Seinfeld*, the star of her own sitcom *Alright Already*, and a judge on the new *Star Search*.

LeMaire has appeared on the *Tonight Show* and Comedy Central.

Jay Leno is host of NBC's Emmy Award-winning and top-rated *Tonight Show*. Leno has also written a number of best-selling books.

David Letterman is the host of CBS's Emmy Award-winning *Late Show*.

Sam Levenson was a beloved American humorist whose books include *In One Era and Out the Other*, and *You Don't Have to Be in Who's Who to Know What's What*.

In addition to his numerous HBO specials, comedian **Richard Lewis** has starred in the critically acclaimed sitcom *Curb Your Enthusiasm.* He is also the author of the autobiographical book *The OTHER Great Depression.*
    Web site: richardlewisonline.com

Daniel Liebert is a best-selling bumper sticker writer ("Jesus is Coming — Look Busy") who has segued into performing comedy at the Comic Strip, Stand-up NY, Caroline's, and numerous more ephemeral venues.
    Contact: dliebert@msn.com

Wendy Liebman has appeared on the *Tonight Show,* in her own HBO comedy special, and won an American Comedy Award.
    Web site: wendyliebman.com

Dino Londis is a comedian and also author of the essays "How to Buy a Dirty Magazine with a Clear Conscience" and "How to be an Asshole."

Jason Love is a comedian whose cartoon *Snapshots* has garnered a worldwide audience through syndication in 32 newspapers, dozens of magazines, 500 Web sites, and a line of greeting cards.
    Web site: jasonlove.com

Hellura Lyle is a Los Angeles-based comedian and domestic violence peer counselor who performs on the CD *Stand-up Comics Take a Stand Against Domestic Violence.*

In a career that spanned 50 years, **Moms Mabley**'s comedy performances include appearances at The Cotton Club, the Apollo Theater, and Carnegie Hall. She recorded nine very popular comedy albums for Chess Records in the 1960s.

Comedian **Mike MacDonald** has starred in three Showtime and CBS specials including *Mike MacDonald: On Target.*

Comedian and actor **Norm Macdonald** has showcased his wry smirk as a featured player on *Saturday Night Live*, followed by the eponymous smirk sitcom *Norm*.

Bill Maher is the host of HBO's *Real Time with Bill Maher*. Who'd a thunk it?
Web site: billmaher.tv

Steve Martin is a comedian who has starred in, written and directed several comedy films, including *The Jerk* and *Bowfinger*.
Web site: stevemartin.com

Comedian **Monique Marvez**'s signature raunchy wit and sexualized sarcasm is showcased on her CD, *Built for Comfort*.
Web site: moniquemarvez.com

Jackie Mason is a forty-year comedy veteran, and the star of several one-man Broadway shows, including *The World According to Me*.
Web site: jackiemason.com

Sabrina Matthews has been featured on Comedy Central's *Out There in Hollywood* as well as in her own Comedy Central special. She has also preformed at the Montreal Just for Laughs Festival.
Web site: sabrinamatthews.com

Comedian **Denise McCanles** is also a reporter for LesbiaNation and has appeared on the syndicated TV show *Night Stand*.

Comedian and humor writer **Laurie McDermott** has performed all over Australia, London and New Zealand. Laurie has been seen in dozens of commercials and international television shows, is a humor columnist for *Bride Magazine*, and is the author of the book *CEO of the House*.
Web site: lauriemcdermott.com

Brian McKim is a writer and a stand-up comic who is also the editor and publisher of the Web site: sheckymagazine.com

Comedian **Donal McLysaght** has performed at the Improv, at charity benefits, and everywhere in between.
  Contact: dak01@alltel.net

Comedian **Kevin Meaney** has two of his own HBO specials to his credit. He has made more than a dozen appearances on the *Tonight Show with Jay Leno*, won an Emmy Award for the PBS series *Comedy Night*, and made his film debut in *Big*.
  Web site: kevinmeaney.com

Comedian **John Mendoza** has appeared on the *Tonight Show* and was one of Showtime's *Pair of Jokers*. He has also produced and starred in the sitcom *The Second Half.*

Felicia Michaels has won an American Comedy Award and has released her own CD *Lewd Awakenings*.
  Web site: feliciamichaels.com

Cathryn Michon is a stand-up comedian who has been featured at the Montreal Comedy Festival. Cathryn has also written for a number of TV series, and is author of the books *The Grrl Genius Guide to Life*, and *The Grrl Genius Guide to Sex.*
  Web site: grrlgenius.com

Comedian **Beverly Mickins** has appeared on Lifetime's *Girls Night Out, Thirtysomething*, and in the movie *Steel and Lace*.

Bette Midler is one on the world's best-loved and most versatile entertainers. She has received Emmys, Tonys and American Comedy Awards, and appeared in the movies *Beaches* and *The First Wives Club.*
  Web site: bettemidler.com

Comedian **Dennis Miller** is the possessor of a God-given sarcasm and the star of CNBC's *Dennis Miller* and HBO's long-running show *Dennis Miller Live.*

During a three-decade comedy career, comedian **George Miller** was a frequent guest on national television talk shows, including *Late Night with David Letterman.*

Comedian **Larry Miller** is featured in both *Nutty Professor* movies and on the sitcoms *Mad About You, My Wife and Kids*, and *8 Simple Rules.*

Comedian **Lynda Montgomery** has appeared on VH1's *Spotlight*, but considers the highlight of her career to be her performance at the 1993 March on Washington in front of an audience of one million people.

Comedian **Maureen Murphy** has appeared on the *Tonight Show* and in the *Girls of the Comedy Store* video.

Steve Neal, a Los Angeles-based comedian, is the writer and performer of the critically-acclaimed, autobiographical one-man show *The Great White Trash Hope.*
    Web site: steveneal.net

Kevin Nealon is a headlining comedian, actor, and one of the longest-running cast members of *Saturday Night Live.*
    Web site: kevinnealon.com

Comedian **Diane Nichols** has been named "a Queen of Comedy" and "the heroine of the 9 to 5 crowd" by *Newsweek.*

Comedian **Bob Nickman** has written for the TV shows *Roseanne, Freaks and Geeks, The Drew Carey show*, and most recently, *According to Jim.*

Conan O'Brien, a former writer for *Saturday Night Live* and *The Simpsons*, is the host of the NBC talk show, *Late Night.*

Despite her humble origins in the Rubber Capital of Akron, Ohio, comedian **Ann Oelschlager** has risen to great success in the City of Angels, where she lives in an apartment building with a swimming pool. Irish comedian **Owen O'Neill** has performed at the Montreal

Comedy Festival, and has been a guest on *Late Night with Conan O'Brien*.

Rob O'Reilly is a Cleveland comedian who has played venues which include the Cleveland Improv and the Comedy Connections.
   Contact: rob84@bu.edu

Christine O'Rourke is a screenwriter and comedian who performs at the Improv in Hollywood.

P.J. O'Rourke is one of America's leading political satirists and best-selling author of ten books, including *Modern Manners* and *Eat the Rich*.
   Web site: pjorourke.com

Comedian **Patton Oswalt** has been seen on *Seinfeld*, and is currently a cast member of CBS's *King of Queens*.
   Web site: pattonoswalt.com

Tamayo Otsuki has performed comedy on the Playboy Channel, *Evening at the Improv*, Showtime's *Comedy Club Network* and in the movie, *Don't Be a Menace to South Central*.

Comedian **Nancy Patterson** has performed at Standford & Son's Comedy House, the Cleveland Improv, Bocanuts in Boca Raton, and at the Cabaret Dada improvisational theater.

Elaine Pelino is a former Texas beauty queen who turned stand-up comedian when she realized, "Wow, getting laughs is like being on a really great date—and I didn't even have to remove my pantyhose."

Mary Pfeiffer is a self-described squeaky-clean comedian.

Comedian **Emo Philips** has appeared on numerous HBO and Showtime specials, as well as in the "Weird" Al Yankovich movie *UHF*.
   Web site: emophilips.com

Comedian **Monica Piper** has won a Golden Globe for her writing on the sitcom *Roseanne*. Her Showtime special, *Monica, Just You*, has been nominated for a Cable ACE award.

Jennifer Post is stand-up comedian and lawyer.

Lewis Ramey is a correspondent on Comedy Central's *The Daily Show*. He has also appeared on the network's *Premium Blend*.

Comedian **Greg Ray** has been seen on *Evening at the Improv*, CNN and *PM Magazine*. He is perhaps best known for holding the watermelon in the Ginsu knife commercials.

Comedian **Caroline Rhea** has starred on *Sabrina the Teenage Witch* and, call out the coincidence police, also has been the host of *The Caroline Rhea Show*.
 Web site: carolinerhea.com

Andi Rhoads is a Los Angeles comedian who has performed at The Improv and the Comedy Store in Hollywood.

Comedian **Billy Riback** has been a producer and writer of the sitcom *Home Improvement*.

Comedian **Adam Richmond** has appeared on Nickelodeon, Fox Sports Net, and several nationally televised commercials. He is also a staff writer for a new animated series in Canada, *Chilly Beach*.
 Contact: gunnyfuy@yahoo.com

Joan Rivers is a comedian whose career stretches over four decades. She also is an actress, talk show host, best-selling author, and fashion commentator with her daughter Melissa.
 Web site: joanrivers.com

Comedian **Denise Munro Robb** has been seen on A&E, Lifetime, Comedy Central and MTV, and is also a political activist who ran for Los Angeles City Council.
Web site: denisemunrorobb.com

Comedian **Ray Romano** is the star of the now-syndicated sitcom, *Everybody Loves Raymond*, and the author of the best-selling book *Everything and a Kite*.
Web site: rayromano.com

Comedian **Janet Rosen** has been featured in the Marshall's Women in Comedy Festival, has written for *Glamour* and other national magazines, and lives and commits comedy in New York City.

Flash Rosenberg is a comedian and cartoonist who has performed at the Toyota Comedy Festival and The Joseph Papp Public Theater. Flash also has been voted Philadelphia's Local Comedian Most Likely to Make You Laugh Until It Hurts, and her cartoons have appeared in *The New York Times*.
Web site: flashrosenberg.com

Comedian **Rita Rudner** has appeared on the *Tonight Show*, has been featured on any number of comedy specials, including her own on HBO, and is author of the books *Naked Beneath My Clothes* and *Tickled Pink*.
Web site: ritafunny.com

Robin Ryan is a Los Angeles-based comedian.

Comedian **Betsy Salkind** has been a writer for the now-syndicated sitcom *Roseanne* and appeared on *Arli$$* and the *Tonight Show*.
Web site: betsysalkind.com

Jim Samuels was a beloved San Francisco-based comedian who died in 1990.

Comedian **Adam Sandler** is a former cast member of NBC's *Saturday Night Live* and the star of a string of comedy movies, including *Happy Gilmore, The Waterboy*, and *The Wedding Singer*.
Web site: adamsandler.com

Comedian **Peter Sasso** performs in comedy clubs and on cruise ships.
Contact: sassopeter@hotmail.com

Comedian **Charisse Savarin** has appeared in *Girls Behaving Badly* on the Oxygen Network and *The Best Damn Sports Show Period*.
Contact: comedy4u@comcast.net

Comedian **Stan Schacter** has performed on the TV shows *Comic Strip Live* and *Evening at the Improv*.

Comedian **Robert Schimmel** has racked up a pair of his own Showtime Specials, recorded the CDs *Robert Schimmel Comes Clean* and *Unprotected* and won the prestigious Best Male Stand-Up Comic award at the American Comedy Awards.
Web site: robertschimmel.com

Comedian **Allan Sherman** became a comedy writer in 1950s TV, on the *Jackie Gleason Show* and as creator and producer of *I've Got a Secret*. While producer of the *Tonight Show* in 1962, songs Sherman had written to entertain his friends at parties were released as a comedy album, *My Son the Folk Singer*, which went to number one on the charts, and were followed by six more comedy records.

Craig Shoemaker's CDs *Shoemaker Meets the Lovemaster* and *Son of the Lovemaster* morphed into writing, directing and starring in his movie *The Lovemaster*. Craig is also the creator of the non-profit foundation LaughterHeals.com.

Lisa Schroeer is pursuing a career in Public Policy while spending her free time enjoying comedy of all sorts.

Comedian **Jerry Seinfeld** helped rethink the sitcom with his eponymous *Seinfeld*, which he created, produced and starred in.

Comedian **Garry Shandling** is the star and creator of *The Larry Sanders Show*.

Craig Sharf is a comedian and comedy writer who has sold material to professional comedians, who include Joan Rivers, and to other comedy outlets such as the TV show *Weinerville*.
   Contact: csharf@yahoo.com

Jeff Shaw is a comedian, humor columnist and staff writer in the Alternative Cards department of Cleveland's American Greetings Corporation.
   Contact: Dork2Dude@aol.com

Comedian **Jimmy Shubert** was featured at the Just for Laughs Montreal Comedy Festival and featured in the movies *GO, Coyote Ugly, The Italian Job*, and *Mr. and Mrs. Smith*. He also has a recurring role on CBS's *King of Queens*.
   Web site: jimmyshubert.com

Sarah Silverman has appeared in the films, *Something About Mary* and *School of Rock*, played a comedy writer on HBO's *Larry Sanders Show*, and has been a comedy writer for *Saturday Night Live*.

Comedian **Traci Skene** is the co-creator, editor and publisher of the Web site: sheckymagazine.com

Bobby Slayton, the self-proclaimed "Pit Bull of Comedy," played Joey Bishop in the HBO original movie *The Rat Pack*, and appeared in the films *Get Shorty, Ed Wood*, and *Wayne's World 2*.
   Web site: bobbyslayton.com

Bob Smith is the first openly gay comedian to appear on the *Tonight Show* as well as star in his own HBO special. Smith is also the author of the books *Way to Go, Smith* and *Openly Bob*.
   Web site: literati.net/Smith/

Comedian **Tracy Smith** has appeared on MTV's *Half Hour Comedy Hour*, and Lifetime's *Girls Night Out*. She has recently released a new CD, *Woman of Mass Destruction*.
   Web site: deartracy.com

Comedian **Margaret Smith** has been awarded an American Comedy Award, and been featured in her own Comedy Central special, and *That '80s Show*.

Comedian **Steve Smith** has amassed over 50 national television appearances and now positions himself exclusively as a corporate and cruise ship entertainer. Smith kills audiences with laughter, but was mercilessly murdered himself in the movies *Nightmare on Elm Street 2* and *Slaughterhouse Rock*. We think it's payback for his father bit.

Carrie Snow is a stand-up comedian who also has been a writer on the first three seasons of the sitcom *Roseanne*.

Comedian **David Spade** has been the star of the sitcom *Just Shoot Me* and his magnum opus, *Lost and Found*. He is currently seen on *8 Simple Rules*.
   Web site: davidspade.com

Comedian **Livia Squires** has appeared on Showtime, has been a finalist in California's Funniest Female contest and appears regularly at the Ice House in Pasadena, CA.
   Web site: roadcomic.com

Comedian **Pam Stone** had a recurring role on the ABC hit series *Coach*, has appeared in her own Showtime Special, and is winner of the Gracie Allen Award from the American Women in Radio and Television for her syndicated radio program *The Pam Stone Show*.

Mark Stiles, originally from Pittsburgh, now lives in the Cleveland area. He performs at various comedy clubs in Northeast Ohio. He has also worked as a TV sports anchor and reporter.

Comedian **Jeff Stilson** has appeared on *Late Night with David Letterman*, and been featured in the fourteenth HBO Young Comedians Show. He has also written for *The Daily Show*, *Politically Incorrect*, and *The Chris Rock Show*.

Strange de Jim has been San Francisco's leading town-fool/masseur since 1972, and is author of a photo history of San Francisco's Castro district published by arcadiapublishing.com.

Comedian **Lisa Sunstedt** has been a featured performer in the Montreal Just for Laughs Festival, and a guest star of *Tracy Takes On*.

Swami X is a legendary New York street comedian.

Comedian **Wanda Sykes** has been the host of Comedy Central's *Premium Blend* and star of her own sitcom *Wanda at Large*. Her first book, *Yeah, I Said It*, was published in 2004.
   Web site: wandasykes.com

Comedian **Greg Travis** has appeared on the TV shows *CSI: Miami* and *JAG*, and in the movies *Man on the Moon* and *Starship Troopers*.
   Web site: gregtravis.com

Jennifer Vally has performed in comedy clubs across the United States and worked as a comedy writer and producer for the *Late, Late Show with Craig Kilborn*, the *Tonight Show* and the Oxygen Network.

Matt Vance has been the morning show producer for *Mick & Allen's Freak Show* on Rock 99 radio Salt Lake City.

Nancy Waite is a member of The Hyena Comedy All Star Troupe.
   Contact: waiten4u2@yahoo.com

Wally Wang is a comedian and an actor who, in his latest performance on the Internet, managed to convince thousands of men that he's actually a 23-year-old blonde. He has also appeared on A&E's *Evening at the Improv*, performs in Las Vegas, wrote the books *Visual Basic For Dummies, Microsoft Office For Dummies*, and publishes a computer humor column in *Boardwatch Magazine*.

Comedian **Marsha Warfield** played bailiff Roz Russell on the sitcom *Night Court* and later joined the cast of *Empty Nest*.

Comedian **Matt Weinhold** won the Seattle Comedy Competition and has appeared on Showtime, MTV, and Comedy Central. He is a regular contributor to the publication *US Weekly*.
    Web site: mattweinhold.com

Comedian **Sheila Wenz** has appeared on the cable channels Lifetime, A&E, and Comedy Central.

Comedian **Suzanne Westenhoefer** is the star of her own HBO special and CDs entitled *Nothing in My Closet but My Clothes* and *I'm Not Cindy Brady*.
    Web site: suzannew.com

Comedian **Basil White** is a weird, scary man-child.
    Web site: basilwhite.com

Comedian **Harland Williams** has been featured in *The Whole Nine Yards, Something About Mary* and *Rocketman* but for the full Harland experience there's his CD *Enter at Your Own Risk*.
    Web site: harlandwilliams.com

Comedian **Robin Williams** received an Academy Award for *Good Will Hunting* and is the star of dozens of movies including *Mrs. Doubtfire* and *Good Morning Vietnam*.
    Web site: robinwilliams.com

Comedian **Eric Wilson** has appeared on the *Tonight Show with Jay Leno*.

Grace White is a middle-aged hippie with a mother who loves her, a father for whom over-eating is an art-form, and a stand-up comedy act like no other. White is a symphony in contradiction, a blur of reluctant energy and a compulsive workaholic entrepreneur who stubbornly maintains her title of World's Laziest Woman.
  Web site: gracewhiteproductions.com

Comedian **Lizz Winstead** is not only the creator of Comedy Central's *The Daily Show* but also — God help us all — *The Man Show*. We forgive her, since she's also helped to create the liberal network Air America Radio.
  Web site: airamericaradio.com

Comedian **Dan Whitney**'s *Larry the Cable Guy* is featured on nearly 200 radio stations nationwide, and has also been seen on Comedy Central's *Blue Collar Comedy*.

Comedian **Wendy Wilkins** has been seen on MTV, Showtime, and HBO's *Mr. Show*.

Comedian **Penny Wiggins** has appeared on TV's *Evening at the Improv* and with the Amazing Jonathan's live Las Vegas show.

Comedian **Anita Wise** has appeared on *Seinfeld*, the *Tonight Show* and at the Montreal Comedy Festival.

UK comedian and actress **Victoria Wood** has appeared on a number of British TV shows and released her own video *As Seen on TV*.

Comedian **Woody Woodbury** has been featured in the movie *For Those Who Think Young* and his early 1960s' comedy albums *Laughing Room* and *Saloonatics*.

Comedian **Fred Wolf** has written the screenplays for and made appearances in the movies *Black Sheep* and *Joe Dirt*, as well as *Saturday Night Live*.

Jim Wyatt is a stand-up comedian, and animation producer of *Garfield* and *The Twisted Tales of Felix the Cat*.

Pamela Yager has appeared on *Saturday Night Live* and Comedy Central's *Stand Up, Stand Up.*
    Web site: home.earthlink.net/~pyager/

Henny Youngman was a comedian and king of the one-liners whose career ranged from vaudeville and the Catskills to Johnny Carson's *Tonight Show.*